BORN

— TO —

FLOURISH

MY JOURNEY TO BECOMING
PANHYPOPITUITARISM STRONG

NANCY HILL

Introduction

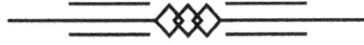

Nancy's book, Born to Flourish, is an enlightening journey from birth to age forty-five, living with panhypopituitarism. It's a comprehensive discussion on growing up with a rare disease and battling adversity at every step, offering a wealth of knowledge and understanding.

If you don't know about panhypopituitarism, it is a rare disease that affects the pituitary gland in the brain. The pituitary gland is the master gland in our body. It controls all the major organs in your body, including the adrenal glands, the thyroid gland, growth hormone, male and female hormones, and much more.

Over the past decade, Nancy has fostered a vibrant community on Facebook, the Congenital Panhypopituitarism group. With 723 members and growing, it's a place where individuals find solace, support, and a sense of belonging. When patients and caregivers join our group, they often express relief at finally finding a home.

Born to Flourish explores Nancy's life in chronological order from the day she was born to her current age of 45. You will learn a lot about the rare disease that she hid for most of her life and the trials and tribulations of what it's like to live with a rare disease.

To learn more about what Nancy is currently up to, visit her website at msnancyhill.com, follow her on Facebook or Instagram using the username msnancyhill.

Table of Contents

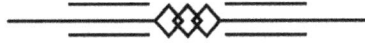

— ◇◆◇ —

CHAPTER 1

Maybe She's Born With It... Maybe It's Panhypopituitarism

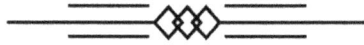

F or as long as I can remember, all I wanted to be was normal. When I was younger, I had this dream life where I didn't have to worry about my rare disease when I went out for an evening. I wanted the freedom to go away spontaneously and not have to think about my medication. The truth is no one ever made me feel like I wasn't normal. I was the only one holding myself back from living a normal life.

I held on to that belief for more than 30 years. I remember many arguments with my mother, with me saying, "I just want to be normal," and with her shouting back, "YOU *ARE* NORMAL! The only difference is that you take medication to survive. You CAN'T live without your medication, Nancy."

I felt like the genie in Aladdin, and my medication bottles were my magic lamp. I was to be stuck with them for life. There was no magical cure to be set free of it. It's a life sentence I wish I never had. That may sound grim, but it was the truth at the time.

My life sentence is to take my medication or feel horrible and die. So, every morning, I wake up and choose to live. I get up, take my medication, and take my shot every day with pride. It's the one task I have to do before I can start my day, even before I put my makeup on. It takes me a couple of hours to feel like myself, but once I do, I'm up and running no matter how tired I am. My medication keeps me going and gives me the energy to do what I have to do on a daily basis.

I'm a 45-year-old woman living with a rare disease that I have had since I was ten days old. That rare disease is called panhypopituitarism. Try to say it three times fast. You may be asking, panhypo, what? Let's break down the word.

Pan = All
Hypo = Deficient
Pituitarism = Of the pituitary gland

The easiest way for me to explain it is that my pituitary gland doesn't work. The pituitary gland is the size of a pea and is located at the base of the brain, at the bridge of the nose, and between the eyes. It is the master gland in the human body that controls the adrenal glands, the thyroid gland, male/female hormones, growth, and more. Since my body doesn't create these hormones on its own, I have to take medications to supplement what it is supposed to create.

The medications I take are:

- **Prednisone** is a steroid that helps keep my adrenal glands going and my heart beating. It keeps me alive in many, many ways.
- **Levothyroxine** - My trusty thyroid medication. It maintains my hypothyroidism, which helps my body produce energy. It also helps with metabolism, skin and nails, bone health, body temperature, digestion, and more.
- **Genotropin** - This is the growth hormone shot I take that regulates fat, muscle, and tissue, allowing my bones to stay strong and regulating my metabolism. Growth hormone also helps with body fat distribution.

- **Estradiol** - This medication comes in a patch form. I change the patch two times a week. It preserves my bones and improves my skin and mood. I feel better with a good dose of my estradiol patch.
- **Mirena IUD** - I also have an IUD that gives my body progesterone to keep my uterus healthy. The Mirena doesn't give me a period.

Without these medications, I would not survive. My body would shut down slowly. I would maybe last for a day or two without them, and then I would go into an adrenal crisis, which you will learn about later in this book.

Living with a rare disease is not easy, no matter who you are or what rare disease you have. Imagine having to take steroids just to live and being questioned about why you were just given three prescriptions for steroids. It's not easy to describe. I've learned to straightforwardly say, "If I don't take my steroids, I will die." This usually leads to multiple jaws hitting the floor, which is a small reward for having to go through rude questions time and time again.

Funnily enough, this just happened to me yesterday. I'm not trying to be mean, but when you're on medications to live, you will do anything to make sure that you can survive. No matter what the drug interactions say, I still need them. I've learned to stand up for myself, especially in the medical world. Taking care of my medical needs is essential. If I don't take care of myself, no one else is going to. They aren't anabolic steroids, just steroids to keep me alive, healthy, and, most importantly, keep me from going into an adrenal crisis.

In this book, you will learn the ups and downs of having panhypopituitarism. This highlights the rollercoaster ride I have been on for 45 years. While this book is a memoir, it's also a journey—a journey on how I learned how to cope with my own illness, how I built a community and found answers to things I was looking for all on my own, and how I found a doctor who cared about my medical care and didn't turn me away just because I didn't need surgery.

Let's get started and dive in. My story starts on March 27, 1980. I was born at 11:37 a.m. I was 7 lbs 9 oz and 19 ½ inches long. I was a beautiful baby with a full head of brown hair. My parents were so proud that their Nancy Patricia Hill had arrived.

I was quickly taken out of the room because my mom needed to rest. They were going to clean me and put me into a bassinet with the other babies; however, within 20 minutes of my birth, the doctors and nurses noticed that I was lethargic and showing no energy. I was given glucose intravenously right away, and they moved me to the ICU. The doctors and nurses hoped that the glucose would help my energy levels. While the glucose helped a little, it didn't solve all my problems.

My mom heard the nurses coming down the hall with the babies and was hoping that I would be one of them. She wasn't able to see me much when I was born, and she was excited to spend time with me. When I didn't arrive, she got a little disappointed, but she figured she would see me later.

At 2:30 p.m., a nurse came in and pulled up a chair to tell my mom there was a problem. The nurse told my mom what happened 20 minutes after I was born. She said I was transferred to the ICU and given glucose. My mom was initially worried that I was diabetic, but the nurse reassured her that I wasn't diabetic, and my blood sugar was low, not high.

My nurse thought I could be hypoglycemic, or I might have an infection. As of that moment, they weren't sure what was going on. They did their best to keep me stabilized until they could get my blood drawn and run some tests. Unlike in hospitals nowadays, blood tests took days to come back in 1980. They also started me on a round of antibiotics to rule out the infection.

In the following days, my family came to visit my mom, and a few family members even took a peek at me in the ICU. They knew I was sick, but they were still all proud of me.. My sister was so happy I was born despite being in the ICU; she couldn't wait to be a big sister.

My mom stayed by my side while she learned everything she could about me and how she could best care for me. They had no idea what was wrong with me - they were just hoping for some answers. She had faith that I would be okay and that we would figure it out no matter what. On March 31, 1980, 3 days after I was born, my mom was released from the hospital, and she went home without me. I don't know what my mother's exact feelings were at this time, but I know it takes so much courage to put your newborn baby's life in someone else's hands.

On April 1, 1980, I was transferred to a bigger hospital called UMASS Medical, now UMASS Memorial Medical School. It's now one of the biggest medical schools in central Massachusetts.

I had to be transferred because I was still lethargic, and no one could get an IV in me. I was taken off the antibiotics because it wasn't an infection, but something more. UMASS Medical had more resources than the hospital where I was born, so it was definitely the right time to move hospitals.

The next day, I was diagnosed with hypothyroidism, which means that my thyroid gland doesn't work on its own. The thyroid is an important part of the body that controls metabolism, growth, and development, calcium regulation, and nervous system function. Besides steroids, this is the second most important medication that I have to take.

On April 15, 1980, I was officially given my second diagnosis of hypopituitarism by a resident at Memorial Hospital in Worcester, MA. Hypopituitarism means that my pituitary gland doesn't function properly.

It wasn't after a CT Scan was done on my brain sometime later that they realized that my pituitary gland didn't function at all. It was torn off and floating on the other side of my brain. They call the non-functioning pituitary gland panhypopituitarism. Since I was born with panhypopituitarism, my case was specifically called congenital panhypopituitarism.

I was released from the hospital on April 30th, 1980. I was happy and healthy, and that's all that mattered. My final diagnosis was hypopituitarism and hypothyroidism.

During the first few months, I did pretty well at home. I was a relatively happy baby, and my parents cared for me as best as possible. My mom was my primary caregiver.

My mom winged it a lot of the time. She listened to what my doctors had to say. There was a time in the beginning when, if I didn't eat on time, I would have a hypoglycemic seizure. I didn't have enough food to nourish myself and hold off until the next feeding. I needed food to keep me from seizing. It was mostly just a guessing game, and they had to check my sugar levels multiple times a day just to make sure they didn't get too low.

My mom went through a lot in the first year of my life. It was rough. She only had two kids - my older sister, Grace, and then myself. She did the best she could with the knowledge she had. My mom always said that she was a student when it came to panhypopituitarism because it was all that she could do—learn from the experts in endocrinology so she could care for me as well as possible. There was no way to find out about Panhypopituitarism. It's not like she could Google it. She had to pay attention to my body and ensure I had all the essentials on time: food, medication, and my growth hormone.

I had the best endocrinologist on the planet. She taught my mother and I so much about my body, and she had a genuine interest in the study of panhypopituitarism. She educated my mother as best as she could on my rare disease.

My endocrinologist wanted to wait for me to stop growing on my own until she started me on Human Growth Hormone.

I started taking Human Growth Hormone on April 1, 1981. A nurse trained my mom on how to give me my growth hormone shot and dilute the powder with saline. My mom practiced giving injections on an orange, which is great for practicing since they say it's quite similar to human skin. I was given my Human Growth Hormone on Mondays, Wednesdays, and Fridays.

The reason why it was called Human Growth Hormone is that it was extracted from pituitary gland cadavers. Pituitary gland cadavers were from deceased humans. The human growth hormone was extracted, processed, purified, and made into a powder. They would put the powder into a vial. The powder was diluted with saline, gently mixed, and injected into the arms and legs with a long needle. Sometimes, the needle was more than an inch long.

Let's just say that I was not a fan of getting shots for a long time, even though I had to take them for me to have a good quality of life. I used to be the baby crying at the doctor's office for blood work. I was stuck with needles throughout my childhood. At under the age of one, I probably resembled a pincushion more than I resembled a baby. I hated shots or anything that was attached to a needle, even though I didn't know better.

During my first year, I had several hospital visits, including a time when I had pneumonia so bad to the point where I was hospitalized. I was in a small hospital (that no longer exists) called Holden Hospital. I now live about a mile and a half from where Holden Hospital used to be. I wasn't holding food down or medication. They gave me amoxicillin to help ease my bilateral pneumonia, meaning the bacterial infection affected both my lungs, and I would just vomit it up.

At one point, I got so bad that my primary doctor, who had just graduated from medical school, had to do what was called a cut down. A cut-down is a procedure that sounds scarier than it is. A cut-down goes beneath the skin to find a vein. My cutdown is located on the right side of my left ankle. You can barely see it now, but for the sake of my readers, I measured it, and it's 2 ½ inches long. I have tiny veins, and I tell anyone doing my blood work that my veins roll. Because just when you think you've got it, you most likely don't.

After the cut-down was done and the IV was inserted, I was transferred to UMASS Medical School until I got out of the ICU, and I was better enough to go back to Holden Hospital. My mother got very upset at the medical staff for not knowing what was wrong with me after they had been called ahead of time about my arrival. She couldn't do anything but watch me get taken care of. My mom doesn't like hospitals to this day, and if I were in the hospital, she would try to get me out as soon as she could. This may sound a bit vague now, but don't worry - you'll learn more about other hospital visits later on in the book.

After my first year, I was pretty stable. I would get sick on and off, but it wasn't nearly as bad as it was for the first year of my life. I was still in and out of the hospital here and there, but not as often. I do have some other hospital visits in the first ten years of my life, but I believe the worst was when I had double pneumonia.

If you want to go deeper into the first year of my life, my mother, Rosemary Southwick, wrote a book called *If They'd Only Listen*. It's about the first year of my life and the struggles she went through dealing with my diagnosis of panhypopituitarism.

As a kid, I was slower developmentally when it came to walking and talking. I got the hang of it eventually and was walking by the time I was 18 months old. My talking was okay, but I had a challenging time speaking in sentences. My grandma taught me how to say "I love you." Or that's what she told me at least. I remember a Hummel or another statue in her home, and she said it was to commemorate me saying, "I love you." I believe I was slower than the average child when walking and talking due to my hospital admissions. Or so we thought. We'll talk about this more in Chapter 9.

I was potty trained rather early, at two and a half, and I did rather well when going to the bathroom by myself. I was still wearing diapers overnight for a while to make sure I had no accidents.

When I turned three, my mom and two other ladies started the process of getting Special Education in my school district so I wouldn't get lost. Special Education was very new in 1983, and my mom wanted to ensure I had the best education I could have, despite my learning disabilities. The ladies, both named Susan, had daughters with learning disabilities. They wanted to ensure that all three of us had a good education despite our physical or learning disabilities.

If I'm being honest, I don't remember much of my childhood until I turned about four or five years old. I'm more relaying what I've been told over the years. I think this could also be because of my hospital admissions. When I used to go into adrenal crises or have hypoglycemic seizures, I wouldn't remember any of it except for waking up and feeling better.

But I was told that when I was four, I had corrective eye surgery because my right eye would cross when I was tired. I don't remember this surgery, but that was my first surgery ever. I haven't had an issue with my eye since.

That same year, I was taken off Human Growth Hormone for three months. The FDA discontinued Human Growth Hormone because, for children, it wasn't exactly safe. Some children were getting Creutzfeldt-Jakob Disease, which was deadly. The FDA didn't know what was coming out of the cadavers, and they wanted to make sure that it was safe for everyone who needed Growth Hormone.

After a while, the FDA approved a synthetic growth hormone called Protropin. I was on Protropin for a while. Since synthetic Growth Hormone was not extracted from cadavers, it was entirely safe for injection.

I was the first in my area to get Synthetic Growth Hormone at five years old. My endocrinologist gave me the first shot an hour before it was released. Once I was on the medication, I took it six days a week. My mom had one day off per week on Sundays to rest.

By the time I turned five, everything started to change. My parents had separated, and my dad had moved out after he cheated on my mom with another woman. My mom was heartbroken, and my sister and I were just as hurt as she was.

My mom and dad didn't argue in front of us because they didn't want to give us trauma later on in our lives, but I did witness a couple of bad arguments as a child. My mom somehow remembers my dad taking the VCR away while we were watching Robin Hood, but I don't remember it at all. Maybe that's why it's still my favorite Disney movie to this day.

As a little bit of a back story on my parents, my dad married my mom at nineteen, not long after she graduated from high school. My grandparents gifted a plot of land to my parents, and they built their house for $25k in 1970. They lived in a trailer for two years while they built our house. My dad worked at my grandparents' chicken farm next door for the next two years until my dad was ready for a change. He started by working as a volunteer firefighter before becoming a cop in town.

They had my sister, Grace, in September of 1976. At some point after that, he became a police officer for a local college in Worcester, Massachusetts. My mom was 25 when she had my sister Grace, and I came 3 ½ years later. She wanted to enjoy her time with my sister and wait until she was old enough to be a big sister.

I had a great life at home. I was a happy child, always smiling and having fun. I loved to play with dolls and Barbies. Despite spending a lot of time in hospitals, I have plenty of fond memories of my childhood, especially when it comes to bedtime routines. Our mom would read us this book every night about the stories of the Bible. I can still remember the book to this day. There was one night that my mom was so impressed by my sister Grace, because she could read the book word for word. She didn't realize until later on that my sister memorized the stories.

Another great memory was when Grace and I got phones for our bedrooms. They were play phones, connected to a wire. It was like the telephone game, except they were phones of the eighties. I believe they were rotary phones. The phone would ring and I would pick it up. I remember my parents getting mad at us because we were supposed to be sleeping. We had a fun childhood.

I was also quite creative during bedtimes. I needed the hallway light on to fall asleep, but it was too bright, so I would wear my Snoopy sunglasses to bed. I did this for so long that I even have photos of me wearing the sunglasses, sound asleep.

I entered kindergarten in September 1985 when I turned five years old. I was a bright and sweet girl who most kids liked. The kids knew I was a little different, but in kindergarten, no one judges. I was slower than the other kids, though. My kindergarten teacher noticed I had some fine motor issues. Fine motor skills involve grasping things like a pencil or cutting with scissors. So, I started with an occupational therapist in kindergarten to help improve my fine motor skills, among other physical issues. My balance was horrible, so she also helped me learn to balance, catch a ball, and more.

You learn the basics in kindergarten, like reading, writing, counting, sharing, playing together, and cognitive thinking. I found this a bit challenging. I think it's because I've always acted a bit younger than my actual age.

I was out sick here and there. I wasn't out all the time, but I was out more than other students were. My kindergarten teacher opted to keep me back a year so I could catch up and be fully ready for first grade. I was a little immature for my age. I don't know why, but I was, and I think I'm still immature for the ripe age of 45. At first, I was disappointed that I couldn't go to first grade, but the extra time in kindergarten helped me a lot, especially going to special ed classes. They helped me with tying my shoes and remembering my phone number, among other little but meaningful things.

I remember working hard because I didn't want to stay back again. That was my biggest fear. So I was so happy when I got my report card, and it said I was going to first grade. I got to see my first-grade classroom, and I was beyond excited to go on my first day. I was sad that the kids in my first year of kindergarten wouldn't be in first grade with me, but it was okay.

Some of the things I narrate may sound simple and childish, but when you grow up with an illness like mine, you do what you can to relate to the other normal children. Of course, I wanted to be exactly like all of them. What happened in the next chapter was a huge part of my wanting to be normal. I don't know why, but that has always been my whole goal in life.

So, welcome aboard to my secret life - to the world of panhypopituitarism and Nancy Hill. I feel weird to say that I'm going public with my rare disease, but it's true. I've never openly talked about living with panhypopituitarism except in Facebook groups, and now I've written a book that talks exclusively about growing up with panhypopituitarism. The only people that know about it need to know about it. This is a vulnerable moment, but I'm happy to share it with you, dear reader. So whenever you're ready, let's dive into the next chapter.

CHAPTER 2

Elementary School

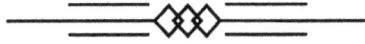

—◇◆◇—

On my first day of first grade, I was excited to meet new friends and learn new things! I loved learning. I enjoyed math, mostly adding and subtracting with blocks, and I was becoming a better reader. I wasn't the best, but I was getting there.

I was still working with my occupational therapist when I started physical therapy, with my gym teacher as my physical therapist. She helped me when I struggled. We would focus on different things depending on the week. Even though my growth hormone was supposed to help me stay strong, I was a bit weaker compared to the other kids. I tried my best in gym class as much as possible, but I always had two left feet. Despite my efforts, both my feet would turn inward. They still do, depending on the day. I made the best out of it and just did what I could.

First grade was excellent for a while. I made some new friends, and I started reading and writing well. I also read aloud okay; however, I was slower than the other children at my grade level. I had special education, and I would occasionally leave class to go out to help me understand certain concepts and reinforce what I had learned in the classroom. I'm pretty sure this frustrated my first-grade teacher just a little bit. I needed the extra help, and she couldn't understand why I couldn't grasp some concepts. Little did we know at this time that I was hearing impaired. We will talk about this much later on in Chapter 9.

Things changed slowly but surely, starting with a day I will never forget. It was the first day that I learned I wasn't allowed to be just a normal kid in my teacher's eyes. I believe this was a form of bullying or gaslighting. It was a fall day—maybe sometime in November. I wore a winter coat and gloves, but there wasn't any snow. A great thing about being the slow kid in first grade is that my peers immensely helped me. I was on the swings, and some kids taught me how to pump my legs. "Nancy, if you want to go higher, you put your legs out as you go up, and as you go down, you put your legs back."

I was just starting to gain momentum when my first-grade teacher stopped me. She asked if I felt okay, and I told her I was fine. She then asked me to visit the nurse to have my temperature taken. My teacher asked the aide if she could bring me to the nurse's office, and I followed.

The aide dropped me off and told the nurse I didn't look well. If I remember correctly, the nurse rinsed the thermometer and put it in mouthwash. I remember she dipped it in something to make it taste better. It was an old-fashioned glass thermometer because there weren't many electronic thermometers then.

The school nurse took my temperature, which was barely elevated at 99.1. I remember the nurse picking up the yellow phone on the wall to call my mom, saying I should be picked up from school. Mom asked to talk to me and asked how I was feeling. When I told her I felt fine, she asked to speak to the nurse, and she said, "If she isn't complaining, send her back to class."

I went back to class for the rest of the day. After I got home, my mom asked me if I was okay. I said I was okay and that I was brought to the nurse's office because I was doing what they asked me to.

I went back to school, and again, at recess, my teacher told me to go to the nurse's office. They measured my temperature, and when the reading came back normal, they didn't call my mom. The recess nurse's office saga happened way longer than it should've. Every day I was in school, it would happen. I would be in the middle of something fun in recess, and they would send me to the nurse's office. I eventually caught on. I would sit on a chair and wait for the nurse to turn around so I could take it out from under my tongue.

I would get caught often because my temperature was extremely low. My normal temperature is lower than the typical 98.6. I believe it's about 98.1. I figured out to keep it just low enough, and as soon as it got around 98.6, I would take it out from under my tongue. I got very good at reading thermometers because I remembered which number the nurse pointed to when I asked what the temperature should be.

Looking back on this time in my life, I was confident that they thought that Panhypopituitarism was similar to AIDS. The AIDS epidemic was significantly real at this time. There were things on TV about it, and no one knew where it came from in my small town. But I was just a child, and I didn't deserve to be treated like I was any different from the other kids.

The daily trip to the nurse's office affected my desire to be outside for a long time. I was always afraid that someone would come and tell me I would have to go back inside and take my temperature. It felt like a daily nightmare even as I got older. I would rather be inside playing with Barbies or reading a book.

One thing especially horrified me. I don't know if it was because my parents were in the process of getting a divorce, and they thought we were poor. One day, as I was getting on the bus, the nurse approached me and asked if she could put something in my backpack to take home. I said, "Sure." She put something heavy in there, but I didn't know what it was. When I got home, my mom pulled out a massive can of tomato soup. I don't know if they thought I was malnourished or if my mom requested it. It was probably the size used at school to feed kids daily in the cafeteria - it was so big it could easily feed 20 people.

When the massive can of tomato soup showed up at my house, my mom wasn't sure what to do. She realized something was happening, but she didn't know the extent of it.

I was treated differently by my first-grade teacher and the school nurse. I was treated like I had the plague, and everyone would catch what I had. I don't know if they just didn't want to deal with me daily because I wasn't the most intelligent first grader in the room. I was getting there slowly but surely, but that didn't matter to them. I was treated like crap daily, and, thinking of it now, it was a form of bullying. They made me feel like I didn't matter or belong. No child should have ever had to go through that, especially not kids like me.

I eventually told my mom what was happening, and she stopped it immediately. She knew I was fine, and there was no reason I couldn't play at recess with my friends. My mom said she wondered why they kept calling her so much and asking if I could be picked up.

At some point in first grade, the school psychologist evaluated me. He would review certain things with me to gauge my mental state. My mom wanted to get me evaluated to make sure I was progressing for my age. I wasn't a fan of the school psychologist. I tried to be the people-pleaser that I was and be as kind as possible. I don't remember much about the meeting with him. I just remember being talked down to, as if I were dumb. I felt that way every time I saw him in school.

When you're evaluated, you're given certain activities to do, like repeating the pattern shown to you with blocks, saying the first thing that comes to mind when you see this photo, etc. I wasn't perfect, but I was seven and struggled a bit with specific tasks. I felt confident that I did as well as I could. But my best wasn't enough. The school psychologist's mind was made up; I would never make it.

At the end of first grade, my mom met with the principal, the school psychologist, the occupational therapist, and my first-grade teacher. I was not in attendance. However, from my paperwork, I remember it as if it were yesterday.

Everyone said I was a lovely girl. I was improving my school work, but I wasn't in the same place as my classmates. My school psychologist told my mom he looked up Panhypopituitarism in a book—that's all we had in those days, books—and said I would be a dwarf because I would never grow, and my brain wouldn't work, so I would NEVER learn. He said I would NEVER graduate from High School either.

My mom and my occupational therapist were dumbfounded. They didn't know what to do. My mom knew that I would grow because of Growth Hormone. She knew I was smart because I could remember a great deal. My nana would call me smart as a whip. My mom never doubted that I could learn and that I was brilliant for my age - she knew I just learned things a little differently.

Looking back, it seems that my school psychologist thought I would be in a home for disabled people, and that I'd probably be drooling on myself at the ripe age of 45. There's no shame in being disabled. Being disabled means so much to the people who are, whether they're mentally, physically, or medically disabled. I have an invisible illness that no one would know about unless I told them. I could always get away with it. People didn't have to know about my Panhypopituitarism unless it was a significant concern. There's shame in assuming that I wouldn't learn anything or grow. I'm 5'4, and I'm writing this book. I may not have graduated from college, but that doesn't mean I'm uneducated.

Toward the end of the meeting, my mom had just about had it. She asked my principal, "Do kids come to school with runny noses?" My elementary school principal said, "Yes, that's why we ask for tissues from the parents." My mom looked at my first-grade teacher, and she and my occupational therapist walked out.

My mom asked that question because my first-grade teacher called her to pick me up from school due to my runny nose. She said no kid in her class had a runny nose except me, so I shouldn't be there. No child was allowed to have a runny nose in her classroom. My mom caught my teacher in a lie at that very moment.

I probably had a cold at the time, went out to recess, and came back to class with a runny nose. It was unfair of my teacher to want to send me home for something every child experiences. And besides, to this day, if I am outside in the cold at all, my nose will run. It's just the way my nose works.

My teachers and administration treated me like I had a contagious disease. Almost as if someone would catch Panhypopituitarism if I sneezed. It wasn't fair, and I didn't deserve it. I deserved to be treated like any other kid. I know it was 1987 - knowledge was limited, and there was no internet to look things up, but they had already made up their minds about me. Why bother with a child when she won't ever learn? Unbeknownst to them, much later, I would learn why I had such a hard time learning.

By second grade, things started to get better. I was finally able to enjoy recess with friends. I was getting the special education I needed: occupational and physical therapy. I was doing well overall. I was meeting new people. Kids knew I was a little different, but they accepted me anyway. I didn't have many friends, but the friends I knew I liked.

I tried my very best to stay on top of my schoolwork. I never thought my second-grade teacher liked me very much. I was taken out of class often, whether for special education to help with specific skills or physical and occupational therapy, and my teacher didn't understand why. I also returned to first grade for math, as I wasn't ready to move on to the next level.

Special Education was relatively new in our area. My special education teacher helped me with their limited knowledge in the 80s. They knew very little about special education at the time. I liked having the extra help because I hadn't learned study skills yet. Memorization was a whole other story. I could memorize things, but it would all become blurry after a while.

In 1988, my parents were officially divorced, and I could tell my mom was relieved. My mom kept our house, and my dad moved in with his girlfriend at the time. He had been living there for a few years at this point. My mom didn't want us to be at my Dad's new house, let alone stay there. My dad and his girlfriend weren't married at the time, and my mom didn't want us to go through the uncertainty of him suddenly having to move out, which eventually happened.

Third grade was a good time in my life. I made some great friends along the way, and I thoroughly enjoyed attending school. The one thing I wasn't too proud of was my third-grade flower press project. Who knew you shouldn't press dandelions and other weeds found around the yard?

I still find it funny at this time in my life. I don't know why I didn't ask for help. I wasn't a girl who would go out in the woods, and since we had a lot of dandelions, I used what we had. My teacher was displeased, but it wasn't the end of the world.

My mom had been working for the new owner who purchased my grandparents' chicken farm. She had already been there for 2 years, tasked with jobs like marketing and making sales calls.

Andy, an old friend of my parents, contacted my mom about a job as a CDL truck driver at the chicken farm. He had a thing for my mom even when my parents were still married. He said if she were ever single, he would marry her.

Andy started coming for coffee to chat with my mom and hang out with my sister and me. They were just friends at this time, even though he kept asking my mom out on dates. My mom wasn't ready to date, so she kept telling him no. Until one day, she said yes. They started dating in June 1989. My mother wasn't your typical dater, though. She wanted a lifetime commitment. She wasn't just going to date Andy - she wanted to get remarried.

In July, my mom, sister, family friends, and I went to my Aunt's house in the Poconos. We loved it there, and we'd spend at least two weeks there every summer if not more. I had the best memories of being there every year. When we left, my mom gave Andy an ultimatum. She said she wasn't going to date him forever. He had a choice to make. If he wanted to be in her life, he'd have to have an engagement ring on her hand when she returned. If there were no engagement ring, their relationship would be over. She wasn't fooling around when it came to dating with 2 kids.

My dad wasn't thrilled that my mom was remarrying. He didn't like that she was moving on so fast with their friend. My Dad knew Andy for as long as my mom knew him; while he liked him, he didn't want my mom to marry him.

But I think it wasn't too fast. They had known each other for over 15 years, and she was ready to get married again. She wanted a great life with someone who understood her and made her happy. It took my dad a few years, but he came around. Eventually, he was happy that we were happy.

On October 7, 1989, Mom and Andy got married. The wedding was a great time. I was a flower girl, and the wedding was at our church, less than a quarter mile from our home. There were around 150 people invited. My mom didn't want a traditional wedding with dancing and drinking, just a celebration with friends, family, and church members.

All of my favorite people from church were present, and it made everything better. Our church was a good-sized community, and it was always a good time. I grew up as an Evangelical Christian, and our pastor would sometimes ramble on for longer than he should.

The reception was more like an after-church fellowship. There was a head table, and I believe there was a champagne toast for Mom and Andy and sparkling cider for everyone else.

After Mom and Andy got married, they went on a honeymoon to Moosehead Lake in Maine. We spent the week with my Nana. She was able to give me my growth hormone shots, so my mom didn't worry about me as much.

Fourth grade was my last year at Hubbardston Center School. We switched classes a lot, and while I liked having different teachers, I had my first male teacher. It was different, and I didn't know what to expect. I didn't think anything would change, and he was a nice guy, but I had never had a male teacher before.

One great thing that I learned during that year was how to ride a bike. I rode it once down a hallway. A lot of people were excited that I had finally been able to do it on my own. Not long after that, my physical therapy stopped. My therapist's main goal was to get me to ride a bike, which finally happened. I never rode a bike again after that one time.

At the end of my fourth-grade year, my mom had another meeting with the special ed teacher and my principal. They no longer thought I was a good fit for the school. I wasn't keeping up as much as they thought I should be. It felt a bit like a throwback to when the school psychologist said I would never learn. They suggested that I go into a one-room classroom. There were kids of all ages there, from first to sixth grade. My best friend, Jen, was in that classroom, which made me feel a little more secure about attending. I knew I wasn't perfect, but it was a bit hard to accept that I didn't belong at the school.

In the end, my mom and I gave it a try. We visited and observed the one-room classroom before the end of the school year. We liked what we saw, and I enjoyed meeting new people. It was a class of 12 or 13 kids. It wasn't overcrowded, and I felt I would succeed there.

We decided I would join the one-room classroom in the upcoming year until I graduated from the sixth grade. We both thought it could be a place where I would thrive.

On the first day of school, a "bus van" picked me up to go to my one-room classroom. Since the students were from all over the five-town district, we didn't go on a regular bus.

This one-room classroom had a name—the Bombay Bicycle Club. It was based on a curriculum called Project Create, which no longer exists, designed to teach students more than just regular reading, writing, and arithmetic. While they also taught the typical topics students should know, the club was more focused on extracurricular activities.

I joined this classroom in the fifth grade when I was eleven. It was enjoyable being there because we did more than just learn the basics; we also had the opportunity to explore and apply our knowledge. We were taught essential life skills like cooking, grocery shopping, counting money, and more. It was a pretty decent structure for most of the kids there. When compared to schools in 2024, it's similar to a homeschool structure, except that we were in an actual school. We weren't always doing extracurricular things. We did our classwork for most of the day, and on some days, we would leave the classroom for art or music classes, depending on the student.

The Bombay Bicycle Club was a fun class. What I liked about it was that it wasn't just about academics. We participated in other extracurricular activities to support our learning. They taught us how to serve others, as well as how to budget and manage money. We would use any money we earned for next week's groceries. We didn't earn a lot, but in 1991, groceries didn't cost much.

Mondays were grocery shopping days - we would go to the local grocery store and buy what we needed. On Tuesdays, we would make soup and salad. On Wednesdays, we served food in the teachers' lounge.

There were always lots of things to do. It was a lot of fun participating in various activities there. We made pies for Thanksgiving and ornaments for Christmas. I had a lot of fun working with my hands. I even remember making mulch for one year. It also taught me that I could do anything I wanted to do. They gave me skills that I never imagined having on my own. It allowed me to understand that I would be okay in this world, that I could be whatever I wanted to be.

Things started to change in my last year at the BBC. My mom wasn't happy that I didn't know multiplication or division, and she found out that I wasn't challenged enough. From her perspective, I wasn't learning anything worthwhile. She didn't like that I was kind of the classroom helper when I was probably one of the smartest kids in the classroom. I got all my work done faster than everyone else. I enjoyed doing different things and helping the other kids. I was learning daily, but it wasn't up to sixth-grade standards. My mom wanted to push me to be normal. Though I was having fun, I agreed. I didn't want to be in a one-room classroom for the rest of my life. I just wanted to be a normal kid. If it weren't for my mom giving me this push, I wouldn't have the average high school experience.

My mom contacted the Special Education teacher who oversaw many of the kids across the hall, and she evaluated me. I was not where I needed to be when I graduated from elementary school. I was not severely behind, but I was definitely lacking in math and science.

My mom shifted into gear and kept me out of the Bombay Bicycle Club as much as possible. Once I got to school, I would go across the hall to the Special Ed teacher's room, and she would help me catch up. If I had a class that my mom got me into, I would go from there. That was my primary classroom. My mom got me into courses that weren't too far over my head, so I could learn more stuff. We worked a lot at home, especially on Math. Thanks to Andy, I tackled my worst enemy— multiplication.

Going into another classroom at any point in the day wasn't easy. I dreaded going into rooms where I didn't know anyone. I felt like someone who didn't belong. I transitioned from a quieter room with 12 or 13 students to one that was double the size. The room was a lot louder than what I was used to. I did not like it when things were loud; it was hard to concentrate often.

I've always liked learning new things. Everything I knew from the one-room classroom was new. I wasn't used to being out of one place all day, but I slowly got used to going from class to class. I think this helped make my middle school transition easier.

Towards the end of my time in the Bombay Bicycle Club, I took a tour of my middle school. The middle school and high school were one big building. We had a large school district with five towns from seventh to twelfth grade.

Taking a tour of my middle school with people I didn't know was scary. I hardly knew anyone in my sixth-grade class, only a few who had previously helped with the Special Olympics.

While I knew people from my old school who were still in my district, I was shy and reserved. I wasn't someone who would go up and say "hi" to people. I saw a few girls from my old school who let me sit down with them. They asked where I was going to school now, and I told them I went to school in Barre but still live in Hubbardston. Most of my old elementary school classmates knew there was something different about me. Not in a bad way; they just knew I was different. Most of them liked me regardless. They all got excited when I rode a bike for the first time. They knew I wasn't 100% normal, but they still cheered me on.

At that event, I made a few new friends, some of whom I exchanged phone numbers with to keep in touch over the summer. One girl lived about five minutes away. It was great; I liked seeing my new school and meeting new people. It was a huge school, and it was overwhelming for someone who had only been in one room for the last year and a half. It was very loud, too—almost too noisy for me.

I wasn't happy at my sixth-grade graduation. I had a skin graft surgery to remove a birthmark that was on my finger. The surgeon was concerned that it would grow as I aged, so we removed it. The hardest part was that we were on the bleachers, and I didn't have a good balance. I'm sure I fell or almost fell on my way down to get my diploma. Other students just handed me my sixth-grade diploma. My principal said, "Nancy has a bad arm," or something similar.

Once I was officially out of sixth grade, my mom and Andy started catching me up and getting me to grade level with the help of a family friend who was willing to tutor me over the summer. She helped me make sense of many things. She helped me prepare to go into a classroom and learn new things. My mother went to the school to find out what subjects I was taking and got the books to prepare me. I was as prepared as I could be. I would have to get by without anything else.

I wanted to learn as much as possible and get ahead, so I didn't fall behind in my first year. I was smart, and I knew I was smart, but I just needed a little help.

I made a new best friend that summer and was excited to go into seventh grade with her. We spent many days of that summer doing fun things, going on walks, and listening to music. There wasn't much you could do in the early 90s, so the best thing we could do was listen to music and go for a walk. Of course, we had to check in every once in a while. Life was good, and I was happy. She learned about my obsession with Michael Bolton. I have no idea why I was such a fan of his. I don't think that the typical thirteen-year-old in 1993 liked Michael Bolton. I had a couple of giant posters of him in my room. Looking back, it was a little weird. I still kind of laugh about it to this day—no offense to Michael Bolton at all.

My mom decided not to let me enter middle school with any records. Since my first school administration had judged me so badly, it was time to go into middle school on my own and get a fresh start.

Life gives us many different opportunities to start over, and I needed to enter a place with no preconceived notions about myself. I just needed to show the world who I was, and I was ready for a fresh start. I went in with an IEP and an individualized education plan and was determined to make it through. I knew I could do it. Doing something new is scary, but I knew I would figure it out.

Looking back, entering seventh grade, I was beyond grateful for the opportunity not to have documentation that I had a medical condition. It made me feel comfortable in my own skin. People just got to know me for me.

CHAPTER 3

Middle School

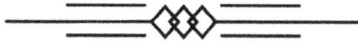

---◇◇◇---

The beginning of seventh grade was an exciting time. I was beyond ready for a fresh start and to be treated like a typical teenager. My mom decided we wouldn't transfer any paperwork from my previous schools. All I would have attached to me was an IEP, which is an Individualized Education Program for my learning disability, and that was it. She let me go independently, and we figured it out from there. If I didn't do well, we would think of something else. If you didn't know, an Individualized Education Program is for kids with learning disabilities. My IEP would allow me to attend a separate classroom and receive extra help when needed. My teachers would stay in touch with my study skills teacher and help me where required.

Quabbin Regional Middle/High School was a middle and high school all rolled into one. Middle School starts in seventh grade and goes through twelfth grade. We spent a lot of time in one building.

At this point, my school was under construction. They were building a new middle school attached to the high school. Our school lacked space during construction, so the district opted for split sessions, which were confusing for everyone involved. The first session started exceptionally early in the morning. School began before 7 a.m., and we were home by 1 p.m. The other session would begin around 10 a.m., and the students would leave school around 4 p.m.

I lived in a 5-town school district, and the split sessions were based on the towns where we lived. The sessions would switch after the Christmas break. So, whichever group had the early morning session would do the later session, and those in the last session would switch to the morning session. It wasn't easy to get the hang of as a kid, but who didn't like going home early, especially when it was getting warm?

My first day was not what I expected. Boarding a loud bus before 7 AM was utterly different from what I thought it would be. I used to ride the "bus van" for the entire fifth and sixth grade, so I was accustomed to being with only 6 or 7 students on a bus. This change was overwhelming, and I could barely hear a coherent sentence. While I was excited to be on a big bus again, it gave me a headache. It was like I went from listening to my quiet thoughts to other noises I wasn't used to. My head felt like it would explode from everything going on all at once.

The day got even more dizzying when I walked into school. I found my homeroom class and sat in my assigned seat. I was with the kids whose last names were from G-H. I met many people from different towns, but I was shy and kept mostly to myself. After homeroom, we went on to our classrooms.

Walking in the hallway felt like entering a foreign land. I barely knew anyone, but I still somehow belonged there. A fresh start wasn't the word. I felt utterly lost in a loud hallway, like I was walking mindlessly and didn't know where I was. I was overwhelmed by the noise. I wasn't used to it, and it gave me another horrible headache.

I got to meet a lot of my teachers that day. My favorite class was chorus, without a doubt. I loved singing, and we had the best chorus teacher on the planet. She allowed us to see a private voice teacher; that was the best news yet! I would finally learn to sing professionally. I was so excited!

This was the start of my journey into the world of music, a world that would become my passion.

I loved to sing, but I'm not sure if I was good at it. It was just something I enjoyed doing. I would've been a happy camper if I had gone to music school as a kid. I was not a fan of academics. I knew how to spell decently, but anything else was hard to understand.

My last class of the day was math—the class I dreaded the most. My teacher introduced new concepts to the students, and I raised my hand. I told my math teacher, "I don't divide." I didn't even know *what* division was because multiplication was the only thing my family and I had ever worked on.

I was a bit anxious at first, but my math teacher was terrific. She taught me that division is multiplication backwards. She helped me make sense of something that I couldn't even understand. She even helped me learn exponents and parentheses—things I wouldn't have been able to comprehend otherwise. I learned PEMDAS, and I loved every moment of it. My math teacher found a way to teach a teenager who knew nothing about math to love math.

I liked school, and it felt great to enjoy it. I had an issue, though. The bus was too loud for me, and I couldn't bear riding it at all. I would come home with a pounding headache every day. I even asked to stay home for a few days because I dreaded going on the bus due to the overwhelming noise. Even if I wanted to, I unfortunately couldn't walk to school, and my mother couldn't drive me as it was a 20-minute trip to get there. I had no choice but to take the bus.

One day, while I was out of school, the bus driver asked Grace, a senior, if it would help if I were picked up first while she was going by our house. The next day, I was bright and early at the end of my driveway. I would go on the whole bus route. It was a long ride, which helped me get used to the noise. I slowly adapted to being on a loud bus, and it eventually got better. By the end of middle school, I did better on the bus, and the noise wasn't as overwhelming.

As time went on, it got a little better each time. I found a friend on the bus and she would sit with me. I was very shy, mostly staying quiet by myself, so having a friend to sit with made the bus rides more bearable.

School also got better as time went on. I felt like I could finally belong and wasn't drowning in a flood of noise. I felt comfortable in my skin, like I knew where I was going, and I didn't feel lost in the sea of kids.

For someone who had come out of a one-room classroom, I was finally thriving at the point where I should've been all along. I worked super hard and tried my best. I did have bullies, but I didn't let them get to me. People not liking me wasn't my problem; it was their problem. And anyways, 90% of the people I had classes with were kind to me, so I didn't bother thinking about those who weren't.

It was great to make friends in school. I didn't feel alone anymore. I made a friend named Lynne early in seventh grade. For the first week or two of seventh grade, we had to stay in our homeroom group for the first half of our lunch, and then we could mingle with our friends.

Lynne and I became fast friends and spent as much time together as possible, mostly during lunchtime. Lynne was much more intelligent than I was. She had the upper-level courses, while I just had the basics, so we didn't get to see each other a lot.

The day had finally come for my first voice lesson. I was giddy with excitement. I thought I was going to sing Mariah Carey or Celine Dion. I also thought I would blow my voice teacher away—that didn't happen, though.

I went to my first voice lesson and was practically bouncing off the walls—excitement wasn't even the right word for what I was feeling. I met my voice teacher by the piano and entered the soundproof room. It was tiny for us, but it had an upright piano, so we could have some privacy. It was perfect for voice lessons.

We started with the vocal warm-ups, and I started singing. I was so happy. My voice teacher was classically trained. She was also an opera singer—and a fabulous one at that. I loved hearing her sing. With a classically trained opera singer, guess what I sang? Opera and songs from musicals—no Mariah Carey or Whitney Houston. I was disappointed, but I was open to learning new songs.

The very first song I sang was "Caro Mio Ben." It became one of my favorite Italian songs of all time. I don't exactly know why. Maybe because it was the only Italian song I knew. I even made new friends who were also taking voice lessons from my voice teacher.

Singing was my passion. It was the only thing I did when I got home from school besides my homework. I lived, ate, and breathed music. I practiced singing just about every chance I could.

That Christmas, I got a keyboard (I think it's also called an electric piano). I loved it. I played it and sang as much as I could. I was so excited that it had its own stand. That was something to be excited about in the early 90s. I had a small keyboard that my dad got me when I was 8 or 9 years old. It didn't have a stand, so I had to use it on a table or my bed. Having a keyboard stand makes singing a lot easier.

On Valentine's Day, our school held a carnation drive (I forgot what it was called, but it was something similar). People paid to get carnations, which were delivered to students instead of candy. I didn't get any carnations, and I was sad. However, towards the end of the homeroom, my sister and her friend came in and gave me roses. I can't remember if it was a dozen split in two packages or two dozen, but I felt special. People didn't understand why I got roses, but I knew why. It was my only year in the same school building as my sister since elementary school, and she wanted to make it memorable for me, which I will remember forever.

I did very well on the honor roll that year and was excited to get to that level. I worked hard to get A's and B's, but I never thought I would see my name on the list. Thinking about where I came from, Bombay Bicycle Club, to being on the honor roll... at that moment, I felt like I could do anything.

Lynne and I went to just about every middle school dance that year. I loved going to school dances. I saw all the friends I made that year, and we had a lot of fun. I even danced a couple of slow dances with some guys who were just friends. I wasn't into guys as much. I believe it was because I wasn't on my female hormones yet. While many girls had boyfriends at this time, I just had male friends. Most of them were acquaintances of Lynne because I was beyond shy.

Grace graduated from High School that year, and it was great.

Towards the end of seventh grade, I was ready to get my period. All the girls had boobs, and I was still flat-chested. I didn't want to look like a little girl anymore. Remember, my body didn't create the hormones for me to have my period on my own. I went to my endocrinologist and asked to get on female hormones, but I was informed that there would be a caveat to getting my period. If I started my female hormones, I would have to go off my growth hormone. I was almost done growing. My endocrinologist urged me to stay on my growth hormone for as long as I could. She said if I stayed on it at least for another year or two, I would be 5'6". I was 5'3¾".

In my 40s, I wish I had listened to her and not considered my period important. I would've killed to be 5'6". It's okay being 5'3 ¾", but I would've liked to be slightly taller. I couldn't wear heels if I wanted to because I would likely fall on the first step. My ankles aren't that strong.

I got my way, and my last growth hormone shot was August 13, 1994. I wanted boobs, and getting taller didn't matter at the time. Luckily, in 2025, it's not one or the other. You can be on growth hormone and get your period, and it doesn't affect anything significant, which is a great thing.

In 1994, the primary purpose of growth hormone was to aid in growth. There was no other purpose besides that, so at the time, getting off of it was just simple. What I learned in my 30s was that when you don't produce growth hormone on your own, you don't have the means to regulate fat, muscle, and more. When you don't take growth hormone, your stomach looks bloated, and it feels weird. Growth hormone also regulates heart health, so it isn't something that should be turned off without much of a second thought.

My boobs didn't grow overnight. I hated being on the female hormones. It took me a few months to even get my period. It wasn't anything special at all. I was so tired of not having boobs that I started getting a bra and stuffing it with tissues. Just about every girl I knew had boobs, or they were coming in. I just wanted to be a normal kid. I didn't want to stand out in life. I wanted to be like everyone else. I didn't want to be weird, but I was.

Eighth grade came around, and Lynne was still my best friend. We spent some time off and on together over the summer. She lived about 30 minutes away, and it was out of the way, so I didn't always get to see her.

I went to my first class and was happy to meet new people. Lynne wasn't in my classes because we had different learning levels. It didn't change our friendship; it made our time together during the day more enjoyable and gave me someone new to see.

I was still taking voice lessons, and we moved on to other Broadway songs. I was a big Broadway fan at this point. My favorite song was "Castle on a Cloud" from Les Misérables. I can't remember if I sang it in voice lessons, but it was my favorite song to sing and play on the keyboard. I loved other Broadway songs such as "You'll Never Walk Alone" from Carousel and "Somewhere" from West Side Story. They were such good songs, and I loved singing them as much as possible.

I would sing for hours at home. It was eat, homework, and then my voice lessons homework. I loved every moment of my voice lessons. By this point, I was familiar with the treble and bass clefs. However, I always had a tough time playing chords along with the melody.

Grace signed up for the Disney work program, and she was hoping she would get in. It would be a great opportunity for her to spend a semester working at Disney World. She would have to be accepted into the program first, but we were very hopeful.

When Grace got the job at Disney (which we knew would happen) in January 1995, she moved to Orlando. She went as a college student and loved it a lot. My dad and his girlfriend at the time drove her down there and got Grace settled in.

When Grace moved to Florida, I moved to her room in the basement. I loved being in that room. Of course, I missed my sister, but it was the best part of her absence. Spending nights in a basement was scary, at first. It was a mostly finished basement with concrete floors and no bathroom. I loved the basement because I had a vast space, well, half of it, at least. The other half of the basement was smaller, and it had a woodstove in it. My cat Noah was my roommate, and he was the best roommate ever.

I was so sad when my sister moved to Florida. I was glad for her, but at the same time, I didn't want her to go. Even though I knew we would talk a lot when we saw each other again, that didn't stop me from missing her. Grace was 3 and 1/2 years older than me (5 years school-wise); we were opposites and didn't have much in common, even so, we got along well.

For my birthday that year, I found out that we were going to visit Grace in Florida. I was thrilled to see my sister and learn about her job. We were going to stay at a timeshare that my mom got for a week from someone, and my aunt was meeting us there. I had never been to Disney World before. I heard about it on TV, of course, and I was so excited to be in this magical place.

Mom, my aunt, and I visited Grace. We were so happy to be in Florida. Grace loved her job. She was a lifeguard at a Disney hotel, and she enjoyed it, from what we could see. She had a good group of friends, which was great for her. I was happy to see my sister happy.

We went to Florida in mid-April when there was a pretty big blizzard at home. We probably got about a foot of snow while we were away. I was just basking in the warm weather, and I loved it so much that I didn't want to leave.

While we were at Disney, we went on so many rides. I went on the Haunted House ride and Splash Mountain. I even did the Tower of Terror at Universal. I hated that ride. It was exhilarating, but the drop made my heart jump out of my chest. I was just so happy to be back with Grace.

After we got back from Florida, things started to change again. My grandpa, my dad's father, got into a bad accident with the Mart van he drove around. This was his job - driving a van for the elderly to ride in. My grandfather would take them to their appointments, Walmart, the grocery store, and other places. He liked his job because it gave him something to do, and it was equally nice since he wasn't in the house driving my grandma crazy all day.

It was April 30th when he got into his accident. I'm not entirely clear on what happened, but I know he was driving and didn't stop exactly. He ended up on someone's front lawn. He was transferred to UMASS Hospital in Worcester, MA. He was in the ICU when he began having liver failure.

We thought that Grandpa would be in the hospital for a short time. I went on weekly hospital visits with my dad, and every week, I hoped he would come home so I could spend time with him at his house. That was not the case.

There was a time I asked my mom if she could tell my dad that I couldn't go to the hospital anymore. It was getting rough on me. I remember seeing a container with his blood in it. I knew it wasn't a good thing.

My grandpa passed away on June 2nd, 1995. He was 77 years old. He had liver failure due to alcoholism. It was a hard time, and my whole family had to go through it together. I was devastated about my grandpa, but I was happy to have my sister back during this time.

I spent a lot of time with my grandparents as a child. I always loved every minute I spent with them. My family had to face hard facts about him after his passing. None of us knew he was a closet alcoholic. He would take a small drink and then go and hide in the garage and drink some more. No one suspected him of drinking as much as he did.

This was the first death that hit me like a ton of bricks. I have many fond memories with my grandpa; he meant a lot to me. I wallowed for a while and it brought me into a depression. It wasn't anything terrible, but I started listening to a lot of sad music.

Not long after we lost my grandpa, I graduated from eighth grade. I was ready to move on to the next phase of my life: high school.

That summer, I found a new recording artist named Jewel. Her album was called Pieces of You. I listened to that CD for hours and hours all summer long. The album's diverse emotions helped alleviate my sad state. My favorite song from that album is "I'm Sensitive." I would listen to that song for hours at a time. I still do as I'm typing this. It's my anthem for life.

My aunt decided to move in with my grandma after my grandpa passed. It was nice to know there was another person with her, and she wasn't alone. She was 70, and she had congestive heart failure, so having someone there helped a lot.

It felt like my world shifted again in just a moment. I went from my grandpa dying to my dad announcing that he was moving to Las Vegas. He had an apartment already lined up. He didn't have a job yet but was still searching for one. Dad said he needed a fresh start, and with my grandpa gone, he didn't have much to worry about anymore.

At this point, my grandma would be good with my aunt, and my dad would be free to go on his merry way. If my aunt hadn't moved in with her, he would've moved in with my grandma and stayed at his job longer. My dad was leaving on my grandma's birthday, September 16th.

It felt like, as soon as I adjusted to one thing, something else started happening.

In August 1995, Mom and I went to drop off Jen (my best friend that I mentioned in the previous chapter) and her sister, Kelly, because they were at our house. We couldn't find our dog, Luke, but we decided he was probably off visiting his girlfriend, a beagle who lived a few houses down and never went into the road.

Jen and Kelly lived close to us, so we were gone for about 5 to 10 minutes. When we returned, someone stopped by our house and asked if we owned a yellow lab/terrier mix. We said yes, and the lady said she had just hit him, and he went off running. She couldn't find him.

It was a terrifying moment. Grace, Mom, and I went to find Luke. We started at our neighbor's house on the right and made our way to the beagle owner's house, where we knew he would be. We found him not far from our house in our neighbor's backyard. He was lying on his side and had labored breathing. Grace and my mom loaded him into the car and took him to the vet.

I waited at home with Andy since they didn't want me to see him be put down if that's what it came down to. That day, Luke was laid to rest, and it was unbelievably hard to cope with the loss of our beloved two-year-old dog. He was the best and most loyal dog. He barely ever left our yard. If he did, it would have been to see his girlfriend. That day was the only day he tried to cross the street, and it didn't go as well as he had wanted.

This year was brutal for me more than words can say. Losing my grandpa and my dog put me in a sadness that I didn't want to hold on to, but I couldn't let go of it. My grandpa's death wasn't my first loss, as I lost my grandfather about 4 years prior. While he was as important to me, this loss hit me harder. I spent a lot of time with my grandma and grandpa; they both meant a great deal to me as a kid.

Death is a funny thing. We know they're no longer in pain, but we still miss them every day. Those family members leave a mark on us because they're essential to us. There were so many memories with my grandpa, and despite his love for alcohol, he was a fantastic person to me up until the moment we lost him. That's how I'll never forget him, despite his flaws. We all have flaws; it's just something he chose to keep secret from his family.

Looking back on these years, I realize I went through a lot at this time. Losing my grandpa was never anything I would have anticipated at this time in my life. It taught me a lot about grief and what it means to lose a family member you're close to.

CHAPTER 4

High School

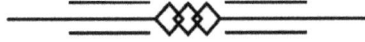

My high school years were among the best years of my life. While I was shy, reserved, and kept to myself, I had my two best friends, Lynne and Kai. They were all I needed in life. I wasn't popular, but most people were kind to me.

Looking back now in my mid-forties, if I could go back and do it all again with everything I know now, the one thing I would change is to learn that I was hearing impaired sooner. You will learn this later in the book, but to make a long story short, according to my otologist, I've had 45% hearing in my right ear and 65% in my left ear my entire life. She said it's like hearing out of a pinhole in both ears. This was one of the reasons I struggled in school, but unfortunately, I outsmarted the hearing tests in elementary school, so we didn't know about it until I was much older.

In September of 1995, I officially started High School. I was excited to be a ninth grader and felt solid friend-wise. Unfortunately, I wasn't taking the same classes as my friends, so we started a notebook and talked about many different things: boys, gossip (rarely), and life. We had codenames for everyone in our notebook. So if anyone ever found it, they wouldn't know who was who. We did this to remain anonymous, so if anyone picked up our notebook, they wouldn't know who we were or who we were talking about. The notebook was black with a smiley face on the cover. I know, it's very nineties. Unfortunately, I lost that notebook ages ago. It was a way to communicate when we couldn't always see each other.

While things were going well in school, life at home was quite the opposite. We lost our dog, Luke, just before I started high school. Grace said it was too sad to be home without him, so she decided to move back to Florida. I was heartbroken that my sister was moving again. We were 3 and 1/2 years apart in age, but due to staying back in kindergarten, we became further apart in school terms. Now it felt like we were being driven further apart by the distance.

Grace got her job back and a place to live, and she flew out on September 16th, which happened to be my grandma's birthday. My dad was moving to Las Vegas on that very same day, and he was driving out with all of his furniture.

I felt like my world was crumbling. Like I had no one on my side to talk to and understand what I was going through. In 4 months, my grandpa died, my dog died, and my sister and my dad moved to different parts of the country. That's a lot for a fifteen-year-old to handle.

I'm not saying that my Mom and Andy weren't supportive—they were. There was just so much going on in my brain that I couldn't comprehend. I was immature for my age and didn't understand why it was happening to me.

I would say that I was depressed at this point in my life. I didn't know it was depression because no one talked about it in the nineties. I felt sad all the time. There was a song by Mariah Carey that I loved, called "Looking In". I was a tragic mess because of everything I had lost, so that song became my anthem that year.

Looking back now, thirty years later, it feels like a distant memory. Life is funny sometimes. We get hurt, but we move on. Grace did eventually move back home about a year later.

I was still taking voice lessons, and my music classes made me happy. I loved to sing. It was my favorite thing to do during the day, and it was the only thing that kept me grounded and fulfilled during those dark times.

The year went by so fast. Before I knew it, I was on my way to becoming a sophomore in High School.

My mom surprised me and told me I could visit Grace in Florida. I was so excited, and I asked if I could bring a friend. So I got my friend Kate, who was Jen's sister. I was very close to both of them. While we don't see each other often, they know I would be there if they needed me.

My first day arriving at Disney World was magical. I had been there before, but I got to see more than I did the last time. We went to Space Mountain, Splash Mountain, Tomorrowland, It's A Small World, The Haunted House, and more. I loved my time at Disney. I saw things I wouldn't have seen if it wasn't for my sister knowing the park as well as she did. My friend, Kate, and I took little excursions to Epcot and the Arcade, where we played Skee-ball while Grace worked.

We also visited Universal, where we rode numerous rides. We did Jaws, The Tower of Terror, Godzilla, and King Kong. We had fun going everywhere, even though I wasn't a fan of scary rides. We even went on a tour of Universal Studios and saw the house where the exterior shots of the Golden Girls were filmed. I found it so cool since it was one of my favorite shows.

Before we knew it, the week was over, and it was time to go home. I felt happier to be home. It was like a small piece of me came back and mended me back together. I felt whole again. While I still felt a lot of sadness, I felt like I had regained some of my sense of self. I felt better overall.

For the rest of the summer, I enjoyed life. I spent as much time as I could at my grandma's house. Whether I was in her pool or not, it was good to spend time with her. My cousins were still very young, so I helped babysit while my aunt was at work. I loved hanging out with my cousins, even though they were a lot younger than me. My aunt was eleven years younger than my dad, so my cousins were thirteen and fifteen years younger than I was.

It was great to help my grandma. My aunt worked all day, so my grandma helped care for my cousins for as long as possible. Grandma was in her early 70s, so caring for two kids under three was a lot for her.

I also hung out with my friends as much as I could that summer. I spent time with Jen and Kate, who lived locally, and Lynne, who lived a little further away. The good thing was that I had voice lessons right down the street from Lynne's house. My mom would drop me off a few times during the summer so we could spend some time together. It got complicated when people lived further away. There wasn't any texting yet, and long-distance calling cost a decent amount of money, so you couldn't stay on the phone all day unless it was off-peak hours, when we didn't have to pay to talk on the phone. Lynne only lived about 30 minutes away, but it was still considered a long-distance call. Anything out of our area code was long-distance.

Summer came and went, and it was time to start tenth grade. I was so excited to be a sophomore. In two more years, I would be out of high school. I was still timid and kept mostly to myself. The exciting thing was that Kai and I were sharing a locker, so I could see her even more often. We decided that Lynne could share the same locker since we were all friends. It was a great arrangement that worked well for us that year.

My voice teacher moved away, so my mom searched for a new one. She learned that a local college offered private voice lessons, so my mom signed me up as soon as possible. I went to the local college for over a year, and I loved every moment of it. The first song she introduced me to was "Caro Mio Ben." I think it's an initiation song for singers.

I sang a lot of the same songs. I had to accept that I would have to sing classical music if I wanted professional voice lessons. I could sing what I wanted at home. I was learning from a college professor, and I was so excited.

I learned how to hone my skills and my range. I was a soprano, and I loved my soprano voice. It felt like an honor to be a soprano back in the day. I took voice lessons every week for over a year, and my mom was never billed for them.

One day, Lynne and I were talking between classes. She told me about a one-act play she was participating in with the rest of our classmates and asked if I wanted to join her to do something fun together. The one-act play was acted out for the whole school and parents, and there would be a vote. It was rigged, and the seniors always came out on top. I thought it would be fun, so Lynne signed me up to take part in our class's one-act play.

My class advisor asked who I was and if I was even a part of the 1999 class. Lynne said, "Yes, she's my best friend." My class advisor was shocked that she didn't know who I was and wanted to be introduced to me as soon as possible. She knew our entire class but didn't know me. I didn't mind - she was the nicest woman ever.

Our other advisor was just as fantastic. I felt lucky to have such great class advisors who cared about us. Although many classes weren't as close-knit, our class advisors brought us together and involved shy people like me in every aspect of our class. I also found out later that my class advisor didn't know who I was because when everyone else was taking her class, I was in special education, receiving extra help with my classes.

It felt great to start getting involved in my class and getting to know everyone. We didn't win the One-Act Play contest; the seniors won it again that year. At the end of our one-act play, we ended it with Prince's Song 1999, the year we graduated. It was great to be up there with my classmates, even though I was more of a stagehand than an actor in the one-act play. I was okay with that since I didn't want to mess up. It still felt good to be involved.

On March 27, 1997, I turned seventeen. For my birthday, I received a rolling suitcase and the news that my grandma, Grace, and I would be seeing my dad in Las Vegas. I was so happy. I missed my dad a lot, and seeing his apartment would be great. He lived right off the strip on Flamingo Road. We went during the April vacation. I can't remember if Grace was living back at home at this point or not.

Flying into Las Vegas was one of the most incredible experiences I've ever had. You flew right into the lights, and we took it all in. Grace was twenty-one, so she could gamble, but I couldn't even be near the slot machines. Luckily for me, my dad wanted to do some sightseeing, so we didn't spend much time in the casinos. We typically dropped my grandma off at the casino, and she would spend most of the day there.

On that trip, we did a lot of different things. We went to see the Hoover Dam and even participated in the dam tour. We saw the Red Rock Canyon. We went horseback riding. My horseback ride was a disaster.

Remember, I am clumsy. I needed occupational therapy as a kid just to get by. I could barely walk in a straight line. It's just who I am.

First, my saddle wasn't sitting right, so we had to fix that. I had to get off the horse without breaking every bone. I had no upper or lower body strength. I was around 5'4", but the horse was still too big compared to me. Watching me try to get on a horse with a weak left leg was comical. I needed help to get back up. Then we had to stop again because my horse wouldn't stop peeing. No one wants to be on a horse when it's peeing. It was just a very comical ride. Grace and my dad were making fun of me the whole time. We still laugh about it to this day.

Another fun thing we got to do was see snow on the mountains. We went up to Bear Mountain. The snow was nothing compared to home - it was so different on this mountain. It almost felt like sleet and had a different consistency.

It was great spending time with our dad. My dad was a country guy who lived in a big city. He loved the outskirts of Las Vegas. Though we didn't do any of the fun shows in Las Vegas, we still had a lot of fun. We were able to do something different every day. We even got to see the Coca-Cola and M&M's store.

We were so happy to be home. When I got home, I had a surprise. My mom and Andy got me a car, if that's what you wanted to call it. It was a 1989 Chevy Sprint. I can't remember how many miles it had on it, but it was a great car. If I crashed it, no one cared because it wasn't worth much. Mom and Andy got my car from a friend of theirs for about $250. Several issues came with the car, but since we got it at a low price, we didn't mind.

My car needed a new engine. The owner we bought it from thought he would give my car an oil change, put the oil where the windshield was supposed to go, and put the windshield washer fluid in where the oil belonged. I would drive my car around the yard until I could afford an engine, or it died. It lasted just under a year. We found someone who could put an engine in my car for $700. In 2024, that would be $1341.30. Still, I loved my car. Mom and Andy were working on moving our driveway to the other side of the lawn, so I had this vast circle to drive around until my engine died.

My car didn't have a radio, so I used a radio with a CD player. I drove around and blasted music. I had the best time driving; it felt second nature to me. Getting on the road was a whole different story. I must've driven through my backyard at least 1500 times if not more. I would spend 2 or 3 hours a day driving in my free time. I didn't have my permit yet, but it was still a blast.

Eleventh grade was when I felt like I was myself a little bit more. I didn't feel as depressed at all, which helped.

Lynne and I had music class together, and it was a lot of fun. To be honest, I don't really remember what we did, but we got to play with instruments and do cool things with music the whole time. We got to play with the percussion instruments more and make music whenever possible.

There was a class I didn't like as much, so I requested to be excused from it. My guidance counselor, who used to be a history teacher, helped me conduct an independent study. The class that I was taking was too loud for me, and I had a hard time understanding anything anyone was saying. From what I heard, it was a fun class, but I'd rather be in a library writing history reports on things we read. I'd rather do an independent study than be in a loud room. So, instead of attending the history class I was assigned, I would work on the computer and do my research using the Internet. It was probably my first experience with the Internet, and I greatly enjoyed it.

When junior prom came around, I didn't have a date, and my class advisor asked if I wanted a date. I told her, yes. To be honest, I wasn't a dater, nor was I looking for a boyfriend at the time. I was just not confident in my ability to date anyone at that point in my life. But I didn't want to go to the prom alone.

My class advisor asked if anyone wanted to go to the prom with me, and she was able to find someone who was interested. He called and left a voicemail on our answering machine. I didn't know much about him, but he seemed like a nice enough guy, and my mom knew his mom, so it worked out.

My date was a good guy, but I was beyond shy and didn't say much. I was not a girl who dated at all, nor was I interested in guys. My date, Lynne, and I went to the prom in a town car/limo. It was a lot of fun. We danced and had a good time. My date was respectful and friendly, despite my nervousness. I remember wearing a beautiful, light green dress. I really loved it.

After the prom, the town car dropped my date off at his house. He was going to an after-prom party. I was not a party girl, nor did I drink, so Lynne and I returned to her house. We had other plans.

Our actual plan was to stay in her parents' RV trailer and party and talk all night. We weren't drinkers, so we just had soda, some snacks, and listened to music. It was a lot of fun. We eventually fell asleep; it was a blast.

In the summer of my junior year, I worked at the chicken farm next door to my house. I was not a skilled egg picker, and it wasn't my forte, but I thoroughly enjoyed the people I worked with. It was a good first summer job, but I was definitely glad when it was time to go back to school.

I had an easier senior year.

I had work-study, where I would help the Spanish teacher during the first period, 2-3 days a week, for my entire senior year. The teacher I worked with was friendly and didn't give me a hard time helping him. Mostly, I would just do copies or correct tests. Do I recall any of the Spanish I studied in ninth grade? No, I did not. The only thing I remembered about Spanish class in 9th grade was my Spanish name. My teacher told me my name, Nancy, didn't exist in Spanish, so he would call me Nieve, which meant snow. There is an actual translation for my name, but it's derogatory, which isn't appropriate for teenagers.

There was a lot of fun involved in planning my senior year. My class decided to go to Walt Disney World for our senior trip. We were set to go on vacation the week of April 19, 1999. We spent around $660 per student, and many of my classmates were going. It was going to be so much fun. Lynne, Kai, and I were going to be sharing a room since there had to be at least one eighteen-year-old per room. I was the second-oldest student in our class, and I was going to be nineteen when we went on our trip.

At the same time, we were also planning our senior prom, the first in our high school's history. My class wanted a senior prom because of the location; Mechanics Hall was a beautiful spot for a prom. Mechanics Hall had a beautiful 19th-century look, and it was what we were looking for to end our high school careers with. There was a one-year wait to have our prom there, so we decided as a whole class to have a senior prom. We would be the first class to host one.

The first half of the school year went by so fast. Christmas came and went, and we were starting to get excited about our trip to Walt Disney World. Not long before we went on our journey, we had an informational meeting about our trip, and we found out that Britney Spears, Sister Hazel, and Reel Big Fish would be performing for Grad Night. Grad Night was for high school seniors, and they would open the park from 11 p.m. to 5 a.m. We could then go on rides and do all the fun things we wanted to do in the middle of the night. We also planned to go to Universal, Epcot, and Animal Kingdom while we were there.

We were excited; our upcoming trip to Orlando was all we could discuss. The thought of basking in the sun, exploring Magic Kingdom, Universal, and Animal Kingdom, and staying at the All-Star Hotel filled us with anticipation. We were going during April vacation to ensure we wouldn't miss school. Our teachers were just as thrilled as we were; it was our last adventure as a class.

The day came when we were finally on our way to Walt Disney World. We got up early and headed to the school to get on the coach buses. The bus dropped us off, and we got to our terminal. We were so excited to be heading to Florida.

We got on the plane, and I sat next to Lynne. We were ready to take off. It was Lynne's first time on a plane, and she was a little nervous and prone to motion sickness. We enjoyed listening to music on our CD Walkman and talking throughout the flight. I was thrilled to show my best friend Disney World and have fun exploring all the sights with her and Kai. It was such a good time. I loved going to Disney World. I was fortunate to have had many opportunities to visit Walt Disney World while Grace lived there.

When we arrived and got off the plane, we got on the bus and went to the All-Star Hotel. There, we settled into our rooms and got ready for dinner. We had an easy night to get settled since the next four days would be busy. We had a lot of ground to cover in the next few days. We had choices on where to go, and some people chose to visit locations other than the specific ones and could stay at the hotel.

To be honest, I don't remember a whole lot about this trip, but I remember Grad Night like it was yesterday. I had a great time being out until 5 a.m., having fun with my friends. Seeing Britney Spears before she became very famous was great as well. I didn't stay for her entire set, but she was so close I could reach out and touch her. It was great being able to see bands and dance with the people close to me.

I spent a lot of time with Kai that night. Lynne decided to take off with some other people because Kai and I wanted to go on rides, and Lynne wasn't into going on rides. Space Mountain is still one of the best rides at Magic Kingdom. I don't know if that ride still exists, but I would go on it if it did.

On our trip, I made a couple of good friends. Kai and I took off with Rae and a few of her friends. We explored the Magic Kingdom together for a bit. We saw some Disney Characters and took photos with them. We also had a blast on a few rides.

We also went to Universal and went to the Tower of Terror—my favorite ride. We did a bunch of different rides while we were at Universal. We had fun, met up with our group, and were ready to go home. Going home would be sad, but graduation would come soon, and we were prepared to be out of high school. After we got back from Florida, everything started to get real. It was crunch time.

It was time to get ready to graduate from High School.

I was thrilled to be back home from my trip to Florida and to have my photos developed at Walmart. I couldn't wait to tell my family all about it. Not long after I got home, I discovered my dad was flying back to Massachusetts to see me graduate. I would fly back with him to Las Vegas to spend 2 weeks with him and his girlfriend. I loved his girlfriend. She was the best. We would leave the day after my graduation. I was so excited to spend time in Las Vegas with my dad. He still had to work, but I would figure out something to do while he was at work.

Mother's Day came, and Mom and Andy took off for a ride. I decided to get on the WebTV and check my email. A WebTV is like having the internet, but on your TV. There would be something similar to a cable box that would plug into the phone line. There was an external keyboard that you used to type on. It was the 90s, and computers were costly. It was mostly filled with chain emails. I would get emails from friends and family, but it was early, and only a few people had computers to send emails.

Every once in a while, I would check out what they called chat rooms. Chat rooms were cool because you could meet people from all over the world. Sometimes, the chat rooms were duds, but sometimes they weren't. Since I was going to Las Vegas, I was looking for something to do with my Dad. I stumbled upon this chat room called #LasVegas-Nights! This room had a different vibe. I didn't have to worry too much because I lived in Massachusetts, and I wasn't planning to meet anyone while I was there. It would be cool, though.

I decided to take a further look into this community. I found out that they would do fun things together as a group, such as attending parties, going roller skating, and meeting at interesting places. It sounded like a safe and fun community, and I was welcomed in with open arms. Most people were either my age or in their mid-twenties. Most of the community lived in Las Vegas, but a few stragglers lived out of state here and there.

I don't even remember how I found the #LasVegas-Nights! chat room. It was just a search, and I was a nineteen-year-old who wanted to make new friends. My dad lived there, so I thought I could make new friends there. I was curious about the other side of the country. I've always been curious about how other people live. I've always wondered about how we came up with names for things. Like, why is a cat a cat? Why is my rare disease called panhypopituitarism? How did we come up with these words? What does it all mean? I guess that's just how my brain works.

Before I knew it, it was time for my senior prom. Prom came up so fast. I didn't have a date this year, but I was okay going to prom by myself. The plan was to go to my friend Rae's house, pick up Rae and Erica, and drive to the prom together.

We arrived and parked in the parking garage. We walked across the street and into Mechanics Hall to our last prom. The hall was so beautiful, and we felt so fancy. There was a DJ, and the music was already going. I wore a black dress with silver accents. I had silver chunky heels that Lynne and I both purchased together.

Rae, Erica, and I walked into our prom with excitement. We ate some delicious food and danced the night away. We had so much fun. I danced with classmates and sang along to songs. I was so excited when my new favorite song, Mambo No. 5, came on. The DJ played so many different songs, from rap to great slow songs, and it was so much fun.

Around 11 p.m., Rae, Erica, and I were ready to leave the prom. People were getting together after the prom for a party. We didn't want to go, so we returned to Rae's house. Erica asked if we could stop at her friend's house for a little while, since it was on the way. So we stopped by there for about an hour, dropped Erica off at her house, and returned to Rae's house. I stayed there overnight and headed home the following day.

My last week of high school was a blast. There were fun things set up for the seniors during the week. We had a fun week planned. On our last day, we had a picnic outside and listened to music. After that, the seniors ran through the halls. We hit lockers, ran, and screamed throughout the halls to say sayonara to the other students. The award night was on the Wednesday before graduation. I was awarded $750 for pursuing my interest in music at an academic level.

Before I knew it, high school graduation was here. The night before graduation, I would sing in front of my high school class and their families. I don't even remember singing or what I sang, but everyone seemed to like it. I'm pretty sure I was off the beat a lot. I did not care to remember that performance because I was so nervous; I vaguely recall it being a Celine Dion song.

My whole family was there, and they were so proud of me. My dad couldn't get over how well I sang. I didn't think I did that great, but what do I know? After the evening festivities, seniors had dinner to celebrate our final night. We were so excited to graduate the next day. We could hardly wait for it.

Graduation day finally came! I was in a tan knee-length dress with blue flowers on it. I proudly wore my cap and gown, and the rest of my family joined us for the festivities. It was a beautiful June day, and I was stoked and ready to walk across the stage. My aunt and uncle came up from New Jersey and were able to attend my graduation along with my nana and grandma. I was thrilled that my family was together to celebrate my high school graduation.

When I arrived at school, we were all lining up and preparing to sit down and get on the bleachers. It was great to listen to and watch all my classmates graduate. We were all celebrating and cheering for each other.

A funny thing happened. They mentioned all the teachers from K-12 who were in attendance. A name stood out to me, and I laughed. The person who told my mom I would never graduate from high school was attending *my* high school graduation. I wasn't upset that he was there; I was proud that I had proved him wrong.

CHAPTER 5

Las Vegas Nights

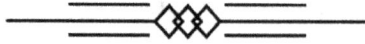

I was excited and proud to be a High School Graduate. I may not have graduated with honors or been a valedictorian, but I did graduate from high school, and I did well enough to do so.

I was ready for the next phase in my life—going to college. I felt grown up and ready to become the person I was meant to be. I didn't know who that was yet—I don't even think I do as a 45-year-old woman.

My dad and I flew to Las Vegas the day after graduating from high school. I was so excited to spend extra time with him. I adored my Dad's girlfriend, Carrie. The only thing I didn't like about being in Las Vegas was that they both smoked, and you were allowed to smoke anywhere except hospitals.

I arrived and settled into my room. My dad had a two-bedroom townhouse with two bathrooms, one of which was just outside my room.

It wasn't my first time in Las Vegas. I loved being in the city because the beautiful mountains were all you could see beyond the strip. I had a lot of fun on this trip. We went to the desert, and I saw Death Valley up close. We walked around and got to explore the grounds. It was so hot out that you needed sunscreen, especially in June. The air was dry, but being outside for more than 10 minutes without sunscreen would burn you to a crisp since the sun was so bright. We also got to see some other deserts around Nevada.

My dad took me shopping at the outlet mall, and I got some new bell-bottom jeans (they were from 1999), a Fossil purse, a Baby-G watch, and, I believe, a pair of sunglasses.

We also went to Madame Tussaud's Wax Museum in Las Vegas. It was so much fun. We saw so many stars as wax figures, which was cool. We saw Elvis, Cher, Brad Pitt, and many more. It was a popular exhibit at the time, and it still is to this day. It was a chance to see a celebrity without actually being in their presence. My dad loved Elvis, so seeing him interact with the wax statue was heartwarming.

One night, while I was in Las Vegas, Dad, Carrie, and I went to see Siegfried & Roy. The show was held at the Mirage in Las Vegas. Before we headed into the show, we went to the Secret Garden, where we could see Siegfried and Roy's White Tigers and Lions. These endangered species were vulnerable and close to extinction. They were so beautiful to see and watch. The lions and tigers were watching us as much as we were watching them.

It was almost time for the show, so we headed towards the theater. As we walked in, someone stopped us and asked if I wanted a signed copy of the program. As far as I know, they were legitimate signatures. It was cool that I had something signed by Siegfried and Roy. The whole show was magical. Watching and seeing what they did with the lions was a great deal of fun. What those lions did was amazing. I never knew they could be trained in that way. The lions were so well-behaved. It was an experience in itself. I was happy to experience it with my dad and Carrie.

Today, whenever I see National Lampoon's Vegas Vacation, I think about that whole experience at Siegfried and Roy. The movie's characters were at a similar show, bringing me back to that night. Magic was common in Las Vegas, and magic with lions was a unique niche they had in the city.

Before I knew it, it was time to head home. My dad and I were already planning my second trip to Vegas. I would stay for another two weeks and was looking forward to it.

It was good to be back in Massachusetts. I was ready to enjoy life and get back into the swing of things. After getting home, I got my first car - a newer one this time. It was a cute Geo Tracker. They gave me $1000 for my Chevy Sprint. It was such a nice car, and it had four-wheel drive.

I would drive around with my friends, and we had a great time. My favorite part was driving the strip on Main St. in Worcester. It was a circle that we would drive around listening to music loudly, hoping we'd get noticed by cute guys. It felt nice to be out of high school, finally.

I spent most nights chatting with my friends in the #LasVegas-Nights chat room. I also made many new friends. I typically spent the hours from 11 p.m. to around 3 a.m. in the chat room. I had a lot of girl and guy friends. I never thought that I would have friends from across the country. It was nice because I could be myself, and no one would care because there was a chance I would never meet them.

It was nice to feel like I belonged somewhere. It's not like I didn't belong in my own life, but having a place where people didn't know who I was made life a little easier. This makes me feel like a catfish, but I enjoyed creating relationships and friendships with people across the country. I felt normal for once.

I felt like I could be a human, and no one knew me besides my name. My name was Nanci on my WebTV, but some people liked to call me Angel. It's how everyone knew me. Since the internet was brand new, and I didn't want to let people know who I was, I went around with that nickname. It was a little weird, and I don't know what inspired it, but I still like that nickname even though I haven't been called Angel in 25 years.

I returned to Las Vegas in August. It was so great to be with my dad and Carrie again. I missed them. I missed the mountains; they were beautiful. My dad couldn't take many days off, so I just hung out with Carrie while he worked.

My dad and I saw the new Star Wars movie at midnight, which I never thought was possible. In a city that's open 24/7, I guess you can start a movie at midnight. I didn't do a whole lot in Vegas. We had a great time, and Dad took me to dinner a few times down the street.

I spent a lot of time inside since it was so hot. My dad's apartment was starting to feel like a second home to me, and it was nice to spend time there. I was too shy to venture off by myself, and since we weren't close to the strip, the only thing you could do was take a taxi. I wasn't twenty-one yet, so going to the casino wasn't an option. I spent some time on the internet. Not a whole lot of time, though.

The two weeks flew by like nothing. I was so sad to leave. I always cried when I left my dad. We had been getting to know each other, and he meant a lot to me at this point in my life. These trips out to Las Vegas helped us grow closer.

I loved having my dad in my life even though he lived 3,000 miles away. I hoped we could have a good relationship no matter how old I got.

When I got back to Massachusetts, I saw my endocrinologist, and I told her that I wanted to be on a once-a-day steroid. I didn't know if this was even possible, but I was tired of taking my medication 3 times per day.

She got me on prednisone, which was a once-a-day steroid, and I started to feel a little freer from my illness.

Not long after I got home, I started college. I was only in a few basic classes—I think I took reading, math, and English. We tried to ensure I was on the right path regarding my schooling. I did my very best. My concentration was music, even though my community college didn't have a music program.

If I wasn't at school or with friends, I was online late at night talking to my friends in Las Vegas. Most of the time, I was up until 3 or 4 a.m. Las Vegas was 3 hours behind Massachusetts; most people would go online around 7-8 p.m. or around 10-11 p.m.

I don't know how I did it, but I made some fantastic friends across the country. I knew just about everyone in the chat room. It was a fun thing to do. My mom and Andy weren't fond of me being online until the wee hours of the morning, but people didn't get online until later in the day.

The end of 1999 was exciting. Y2K was upon us, and we were ready to determine if the computers would stop working. Because we were in the new millennium, we weren't sure what would happen when we went from 1999 to 2000. The theory was that everything with a date on it, like the TVs and computers, would just turn off and never work again.

I stayed at Lynne's house for New Year's Eve, and we waited until midnight to ensure everything would still work. In the backs of our minds, we knew it would. It was just going from a 9 to a 0; I don't think changing a date would be that hard. Of course, the world didn't shut down, and we were okay. We were all very new to the world of technology. No one knew what would happen. But the TV and the internet were still working, so that's all that mattered.

Cell phones were pretty new, and not many people had them. If the family cell phone worked, then everything was fine. It was unusual for many people to have a cell phone back then. There was typically one cell phone per family, and whoever went the furthest used the cell phone.

I still had plenty of time off from college. We got about a month off, and I wanted to see my dad and Carrie again. I was excited because a few days after I was going to be there, my chat room, #LasVegas-Nights!, had a party coming up at someone's apartment. I was so excited to get to know people.

When I arrived in Las Vegas, my dad picked me up. It was so good to see him and Carrie again. About a day after I got to Vegas, I told my dad about my chat room friends, and he agreed that I could go. He was unsure about it, but if he saw the people picking me up, he'd be okay with me going.

The party day came, and I was ready to go. My friend Evie, her boyfriend, and our friend Jake picked me up. I had met Evie's boyfriend in person before; we went on one date in August when I was in Vegas. He was an okay guy, but it didn't generally work out.

We went to get food, and then we headed to the party. I was VERY shy. Everyone was excited that I was there. It was just finally good to be in a space with these people. I felt safe, and everyone was kind to me. It was my first experience meeting people I knew online.

We were celebrating someone's birthday, so we had a cake. It was just good to be in person with people I never would've met without that chat room. It was weird to put names to faces. Most of us had a nickname that wasn't our name. I just changed my name from Nancy to Nanci. It was different and unique, but I still had my name.

When we introduced ourselves, many of us said our usernames so we would know who was who. Most people knew each other since they had done different and fun activities together, so I was the only newcomer.

We left the party at a decent time. I didn't drink alcohol at all, and they drove me home. The next day, I went to do some fun things with Evie and Jake. We hung out and explored the Circus Circus casino, and we just walked around and had a good time.

It was nice to have fun with people while my dad was at work. It was all purely innocent - we drove around and listened to music in the car.

Evie and Jake eventually dropped me off, and I had dinner with my dad and Carrie. We went to a little Italian restaurant down the street from my dad's house. We had so much fun just hanging out.

A few days before I was supposed to leave, Dad and I did some errands. I felt tired while I was getting ready, so I told my dad I would nap since we weren't going anywhere for a while. About an hour later, my dad found me unconscious on the bed, and he couldn't wake me up. He called Carrie, and they got me to the ER immediately.

Panhypopituitarism is a very different rare disease. If my body doesn't have enough cortisol, it will start to shut down very slowly, and I would go into something called an adrenal crisis.

An adrenal crisis occurs when the adrenal glands don't produce enough cortisol. I take cortisol, also known as steroids, to live, and when my body doesn't produce enough cortisol, it starts to shut down slowly.

Common symptoms of an adrenal crisis are:

- Abdominal pain or flank pain
- Confusion, lack of consciousness, or coma

- Dehydration
- Feeling lightheaded
- Low blood sugar
- And so much more

When I arrived at the hospital, they had to cut my clothes off me. I was still unconscious. They were having a hard time getting an IV in me, and they tried many places. They finally landed on putting a central line in my neck. I remember waking up in the emergency room. I was still out of it, but I was so weak that I couldn't speak.

I knew a little about what panhypopituitarism was, but I was still really clueless. My dad and Carrie had no idea because they were so far removed from my illness, and my mom took care of it all. The doctors and nurses kept saying that my blood sugar was low. They started pumping me with glucose and fluids. This helped a little, but, as you know, it can't solve all my problems. I also had a catheter, so I wouldn't need to go to the bathroom while I was there.

I felt so sick and so weak that I could barely move. They kept telling my parents, because I was over the age of eighteen, that no one could tell them what to do but me. I was so flustered because I barely knew about my diagnosis besides the basics.

At 2 a.m. in Las Vegas, my mom called the nurse's station and talked to my nurse. My mom started telling her about my diagnosis, and she told my mom I was nineteen and considered an adult. My mom said, "She has a medical alert bracelet on her wrist. Did you see it?"

My nurse said, "Oh my God!" and hung up on my mother.

She found my medical alert bracelet. They started giving me hydrocortisone while I was still getting glucose, which was dangerous. I remember the next day telling my mom that they were going to kill me if I didn't get out of there. My mom came up with a plan for me to start refusing medications.

The only thing they could give me was hydrocortisone, and I would refuse the rest. Once I started refusing the medicines, they were a little more eager to get me out of there. The problem was that I was very weak. My mom wanted me home as soon as possible. I got on a flight the next day after being released from the hospital.

Before I left, Carrie helped me take a shower. All I could do was sit there while she helped me clean up. I felt so weak I could barely stand. The thing is, I can't remember how I ended up in an adrenal crisis. I was taking my medication—unless I forgot. Prednisone only needed to be taken once a day and would last through my system for 24 hours. I believe I was on a higher dose than I should've been.

My dad had to get a wheelchair for me to get me to the terminal. He hugged me, and we both cried as I left. I didn't want to be alone, and it was hard while I was on the plane, but the flight attendants kept a good eye on me and ensured I was okay.

I was on a one-way flight and didn't have a layover. When I landed, Mom and Grace were there to welcome me home. Grace and Mom were shocked to see my bruises from the hospital, where they were trying to get an IV in me. I cried as soon as I saw them, and Grace was surprised that I was in a wheelchair. My mom wasn't surprised at all. She got my medication right away. I had already taken my Synthroid, and she got me back on hydrocortisone, so I started feeling a lot better.

When I got home, Mom took photos of the bruises that were all over my body. They weren't little bruises. The one on my neck alone covered half of my neck. I felt so ashamed and didn't want to return to school because of it. I didn't want people to look at me with a massive bruise on my face. We made sure they stayed covered, and I began to feel better slowly. My mom decided to change endocrinologists because I was an adult, and my endocrinologist was pediatric, for children under eighteen.

We changed endocrinologists right before my twentieth birthday, and I got back on growth hormone. That was a change. I had been off growth hormone since I was fourteen, and I was not happy knowing that I would have to take a shot every day again.

My endocrinologist put me on a growth hormone called Humatrope. It was the first injector pen that I ever used. It was terrific, and I didn't need a long needle or anything. I still had to mix it, but I was trained to do so. Humatrope was the first growth hormone shot that my mother didn't have to give me. She watched me the first time I took it and was excited about the new technology. It was completely different from the half-inch needle I had in 1994.

Mom and Andy bought me a mini fridge so that my medication wouldn't have to be stored in our main refrigerator, and I would have easy access to it. Things were finally looking up, and I was happy and thriving, and that's all that mattered. I felt much better being on the growth hormone. I had more energy, and my stomach didn't look weird anymore.

You may be wondering why I chose to take growth hormone. My new endocrinologist said that it would help me. Even though your body stops growing when your bones fuse, there are still benefits to taking growth hormone. It aids in heart and bone health and regulates fat, muscle, and body tissue. It also helps with metabolism and blood sugar levels.

When your body doesn't produce growth hormone, there are some symptoms:

- Reduced sense of well-being
- Anxiety and or depression
- Decreased energy
- Increased body fat
- Decreased muscle tone
- Decreased bone density
- Insulin resistance

Living with panhypopituitarism, I don't have a choice in taking it if I want to live a healthy and sustainable life. I remember having a lot of these symptoms for many years, especially as a teenager. I always wondered why I felt so down and depressed, especially after my grandpa died. This was the answer.

I finally started to thrive and feel better when I remembered to take it. Remembering to take my medication was a whole other thing that we'll get into later.

I felt like my life was finally taking shape. I got a part-time job as a hostess in a restaurant in a small town called Phillipston. I stayed there for about a month. I was paid in cash, and I didn't understand the restaurant's job or layout. I would describe it as an unusual restaurant. Upon further research, I discovered that it was an old horse barn that had been converted into a restaurant. I remembered there was an open pool, but I'm unsure if it was open to the public.

Not too long after, I found a babysitting job in a nearby town. It was a Monday through Friday job, and they had two kids. I loved babysitting those kids. We would play outside and go for walks. The son loved to watch The Wizard of Oz - it was on for so much of the day, especially if it was cold outside. I was still going to school, and the kids' mom worked with me to ensure I could help whenever possible. I was their babysitter for at least a year and a half, if not longer. I don't remember why we went our separate ways. I left on good terms and lost touch with them over the years.

My first car accident ever happened when I was on my way home from meeting my friend for breakfast. My mom advised me not to go because of the bad weather, and I went anyway.

It was raining, and I was in my Geo Tracker on the highway. On my way home, I hit a puddle on the side of the highway and hydroplaned. I believe I was passing an oil truck. I was going about 65 in a 55, which, considering my car's top speed is 85, was pretty fast.

I crashed into some trees and I was injured with cuts and scrapes. No one else was hurt, which was a miracle. My elbow went through the window of my Geo Tracker, which was similar to a Jeep. My car was totaled, and I was banged up.

I was stitched up at the emergency room afterward. My mom was upset with me. My whole family was. I had only had my license for about a year and a half and had no idea how to use it responsibly. Getting into an accident like that made me realize that I need to be cautious when driving in the rain and not always drive at top speed.

As the fall arrived, I went back to school. I remember having pain in my elbow. I didn't think much of it until the pain got unbearable. It hurt to drive, and as time went on, the pain got worse and worse. It felt like there was glass stuck in my arm. I didn't know what it was.

My mom got an appointment with an orthopedic surgeon to get a second opinion. The surgeon did an MRI and found out there were four pieces of glass in my elbow from my accident. We scheduled surgery, and he took the glass out of my elbow. I kept four little pieces of glass in my arm for three months.

After my surgery, I started to feel a lot better, and I could drive again without having pain. I spent a lot of time with my friends and just enjoyed living life to the fullest.

I was still figuring out what I wanted to do in my life. I had a variety of classes that I enjoyed. My favorite class at that time was poetry. I took poetry for as long as I could. It was a night class once a week from 6-9 pm. I made a lot of great friends in that course, and I did a couple of poetry readings. I think I did ok at poetry, but overall, it wasn't my forte. My other classmates wrote better poetry than I did. Unfortunately, I discarded all of that years ago, so I no longer have any of the poems I wrote.

The one thing I know is that I love to write. It helped me stay creative, and I loved doing any creative thing that I could.

As time went on, I had this idea for a business that I never opened. It was called Entertainment Emporium. It was different from what you would think in today's world. They have these types of things now, where you can go mini-golfing and bowling within a few feet of each other.

This idea was more for the creative side of who I am.

The Entertainment Emporium would be based in a two-story building, open from 9 a.m. to 2 a.m. During the day, it was an internet cafe - you could have coffee and sit at the computer and check email or go on Myspace. There would also be classrooms where people could take a class or learn something new. At night, it was a bar where you could sing karaoke or a band could play. Bands could sell their merch and CDs in our store, where we could sell books and all types of CDs. The Entertainment Emporium was a vast idea with numerous plans.

My imagination for creating things like this was incredible. I had everything ready to go, from signs to Karaoke challenges. It was just something I did to keep myself busy. Maybe I would open it one day, but it was just fun to dream and imagine opening this humongous business that was all my own.

In 2025, this wouldn't fit into the scope of where these things are. We walk around with computers in our hands all day long that can do everything we can imagine and more.

I've always been able to see the bigger picture and create something out of nothing. My panhypopituitarism brain has so much creativity that there are days in my mid-forties when I just look at what I want to create next.

The incredible thing about this is that I can create something out of nothing, especially when it comes to websites or business ideas.

Thinking up the Entertainment Emporium gave me something I would've never dreamed of creating. Even though it didn't turn into a business, it gave me insight that I could be anyone I wanted. I could be a business mogul if I wanted to. I'm not that person today, but I still have the rest of my life to figure it out.

CHAPTER 6

From Super Fan to Wonder Woman

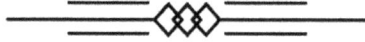

———⟨◇◇◇⟩———

In 2003, I began working part-time at a local car dealership. I worked from 5 to 8 p.m. a few days a week and cashed out people who had their cars serviced during the day but were late to pick up their vehicles. I enjoyed the job; it was slow during the evenings, so it wasn't as bad.

I also started volunteering for Wired Safety, which works to combat cyberbullying in schools and other programs. I loved working with kids in a web-based format. I had no idea what I was doing, but it was incredibly fun to help new schools get started with Wired Safety and their Teen Angels program. I learned very quickly and worked closely with our volunteer coordinator. I had a blast doing it, even though it was with people I never knew or planned on meeting. It was purely a volunteer-based non-profit. I loved working with volunteers and made many friends around the world. We all went by anonymous nicknames.

I loved it because it gave me a purpose besides being a secretary—no offense to those working in that field. I needed more for my life than a regular job. I've always known that. Not that I was better than an ordinary job, but working a 40-hour week was never for me.

Multi-passionate isn't quite the word, but my mind always kept me busy. I don't like to watch TV just for the sake of watching it. I always have to be doing something with my hands, whether playing a game or working on my computer. I loved doing projects, coloring, or engaging in other activities. However, in my 40s, I still can't engage in mindless activities. I'd rather be doing something constructive.

I was also passionate about attending live music performances. I loved listening to live music, going out, talking to musicians, and having fun dancing. I made friends with people in a couple of bands, and it was good just to have fun and get to know people when they had time to talk. I would often hang out with bands for most of the night. I was known as a "super fan" of one band. I had an appreciation for all types of genres. I would go out 2 or 3 nights a week, depending on whether a band was nearby. Kai would come some nights, and we'd have a blast.

My favorite band was called Violet Nine—a real band name. They were a band based in Boston and would occasionally come to Central Mass. They had a unique sound that wasn't anything easy to describe. They were nice guys; hanging out with them was fun when they weren't busy playing music. I didn't date anyone in the band. I just liked listening and dancing to their music. The dancing part was my favorite, even though I don't think I had any real dance rhythm. I would see other bands too, but I simply adored Violet Nine. I was happy and felt good to be back in the music scene.

By the time I turned 25, I was still attending school, but I had transitioned to a four-year institution instead of just my local community college. My issue was that I had so many interests that I couldn't keep my sights long on any particular subject. I loved business, writing, and a bunch of different things. I guess that would mean that I'm multi-passionate.

I loved the idea of being a teacher, so I decided to make that my career. Oh boy, was I wrong.

Teaching was not my strong suit. I liked working with the kids, but the thought of getting up there and teaching all day was not what I wanted to do. My initial path was to become a high school English teacher because I loved all of my English teachers, and they made the world a better place for me. I did pretty well, but it wasn't my passion. Additionally, an event occurred that slightly altered the trajectory of my education.

I broke my fibula while I was walking to class. I slipped in the professor's parking lot, and it hurt badly. I struggled to find the campus police telephone number, and they immediately dispatched the ambulance. I told the ambulance that I needed steroids because I have adrenal insufficiency, which again means my body doesn't create the necessary steroids for stressful situations like a broken bone. They did get me steroids not long after I got to the hospital. My mom was Christmas shopping with friends, so Andy and Grace picked me up. With a broken fibula and my lack of good balance, using crutches was not fun for me.

The hospital put me in a boot and gave me Vicodin. It hurt so bad that I could barely walk on my feet. My mom decided we should get a second opinion, so we found a good orthopedic surgeon. They thought that I might need surgery, which I was not looking forward to at all. The boot cost us $600 because my insurance wouldn't cover it. This annoyed my mom, who wasn't happy with the other hospital for giving me a boot in the first place.

We drove to Worcester for my orthopedic surgeon's appointment, and it was not fun to be in a car again. When we arrived at the hospital, Mom put me in a wheelchair because the crutches and I didn't work well together. She brought me to my doctor's appointment because I couldn't drive myself. My mom was my advocate for me in every way at this time.

My doctor said that we don't have to operate, and it should just heal on its own. My mom asked if we could have a cast because I was not doing very well in the boot or with the crutches. They put a cast on and got me a walker that I would use like crutches. These gave me more stability.

I took a six-week leave of absence from school. I also took some time off from the car dealership since I couldn't drive. Luckily, it was close to Christmas break, so I had a decent amount of time off from school.

I lived in my parents' basement, but since I couldn't hop up and down the stairs, they wanted me to stay upstairs so I could get around more easily. I was so clumsy, I wasn't going to be able to climb the stairs anyway. I wanted to be in my room though, so I decided I would get on the floor and crawl up and down the stairs with my butt. I'd crawl butt first to my chair and sit there for the day. I don't remember how I got up, but I was able to do it. If I had to go to the bathroom or eat food, I would use my walker. I wish knee scooters were an accessible thing back in 2005. Though, knowing my clumsy self, that wouldn't be a good idea either.

The problem in the beginning was that the Vicodin was making me extremely tired, and when I wasn't exhausted, I was throwing up. I opted to just live with the pain and hope that it would get better over time.

I was in a cast for about six weeks, and I wore the boot for another two weeks. I was able to start the new semester, and after consulting with my advisor, we decided that I would switch to another major for a while. I still wanted to be an English major, so I opted for a creative writing major. I was able to finish my finals when I got back, and I did okay. I was glad that I changed my major because teaching didn't feel like a good fit for me.

We were working on short stories at one point in my new major, and I had a lot of fun. I had never thought of writing stories before. I had written poetry, but writing stories was a different experience. You were able to be as creative as you could with writing a book or just a short story. Things were open when I wrote. I had a hard time with character development, and there wasn't much information about it then, as there is now, but it was an enjoyable experience.

As time went on in school, I struggled to concentrate on the more boring subjects. I wanted to pass all my classes, but I had little to no interest in some of them. Sometimes I just wouldn't go to class.

I don't know why I didn't just drop the classes. I just got bored with particular subjects, and to me, they weren't worth all my full attention. I lost interest in some subjects relatively quickly. I didn't know what was going on with me. I just wanted to succeed at something in life, but I felt like I was doing the opposite. The weird part was that I was having a more challenging time when the classes were louder or when too many people were talking at once. We will get back to this much later, though.

There was a point where I started to feel depressed. Even though I had friends and went out a lot, I didn't know what I wanted to do with my life. I wanted more than what I was given, more than panhypopituitarism.

There were so many unanswered questions, and I didn't have an outlet to ask people about my rare disease. I could ask my mom and my doctor, but at this point, it just wasn't enough for me. I wanted someone similar to me. Someone else who was born with my disease, with whom I could ask questions. I didn't have that, and it hurt.

One burning question that I wanted to know about was if I could have children. It wasn't a huge priority in my life since I wasn't married or dating anyone seriously. I got brave and went to a gynecologist who specializes in endocrinology disorders. I was twenty-seven when I first went in. It was my first time seeing a gynecologist, and I was beyond scared. Only my PCP and my endocrinologist had dealt with managing my female hormones before. Going to a gynecologist was new, and I was nervous. I hated getting pap smears, and I knew I would have to get them to find out if I could have kids or not.

I met with the reproductive endocrinologist. He told me that the only way for us to find out if I could have kids was if he ran some tests and did an ultrasound. The ultrasound technician informed me that everything appeared to be in order. I discovered that I could be a mother if I chose to be. My blood tests came back fine.

My reproductive endocrinologist told me that I could indeed have children. The older I got, the higher the risk of a pregnancy would be, but this office was willing to make it happen if I got married by the time I was thirty-five. I could have children later, but they wanted to ensure that I wouldn't be at a high risk.

They didn't want to wait too long for me to have kids because of my panhypopituitarism. I took steroids, and I would have to go down on that if not entirely off, because it would hurt the fetus, which can be dangerous for me to go through for nine months.

I would most likely have to get pregnant through IVF, and that would cost thousands of dollars that I didn't have. I also didn't have anyone that I was even close to marrying at this point in my life. It was honestly just a question I had wanted answered for so long that their answer, "Yes, we can try when and if the time comes," made me extremely happy. I was just pleased to find out that I could have children if I wanted them.

I had a spring in my step for a while, knowing that I could have children if I wanted them. There was a 3% chance I could have kids naturally. I didn't think it would happen because I was on female hormones, and that was the only way my body was working in the way it should.

I was not in a position to have kids. I was single, I dated, but no one struck my interest long enough to date long-term and be happy for the rest of my life. I did not want to be a single mother. I struggled enough with panhypopituitarism, never mind bringing a child into this world by myself. I was happy to have had the opportunity to have kids, if that had been my choice.

I would have to wait and see if it was in the cards. If it was, wonderful. If not, I was happy just knowing that I had the opportunity to be a mother.

Now, let's get back to my story.

In May 2008, my mom discussed a self-help program with my cousin. My cousin, Kristina, thought it would be beneficial for me to take one class and see if I gained anything from it. There were more classes, but we would just start there and see if I wanted to continue. It was a three-class program: there was Trek, Everest, and leadership. I would take Trek and see if I wanted to move on to Everest and beyond.

Kristina and I interviewed to assess my current situation and see what I wanted to achieve in life. She had me write out everything and told me to keep the paper and bring it with me on my trip.

As the days drew nearer to going to Florida, I was so excited and had everything I could ever need packed in my suitcase. I packed way too early, just to make sure I had everything. I was ready to change my life and feel like a new person. I was tired of being depressed and just not happy in general.

I was thrilled to visit Fort Myers, Florida, and see Kristina. When I landed, I was anxious that I wasn't going to find my cousin and reach my destination. The airport I flew into was a very easy airport to navigate, so at least I didn't have to worry about getting lost.

Kristina told me how much the program helped her gain perspective and make many friends. She was excited and hopeful that I would gain a lot from this course. She told me to trust the process and that all would be okay.

Friday came, and we went to the beach for a bit. I was in love. I had never seen such a beautiful beach in my life. The sand was so soft that it felt like walking on a cloud. I've never felt more in love with a place than I did with Fort Myers. It was everything I wanted in my life.

On my first night, I gained a decent understanding of myself and learned how to maintain a positive outlook. I met many wonderful people and learned that I was enough. I began to feel happier.

The second and third days felt life-changing. I had started peeling my layers off little by little. I learned that I get to live every day to the fullest. It's my life and my choice, no matter what. One sentence I can remember out of that whole weekend is I GET TO LIVE. No one can decide that for me.

By the end of the weekend, my mindset had shifted, and I started thinking at a whole new level. It was a massive change for me. We were told at graduation that once you graduate from Trek, you can always come back on Friday night for the mind set shift. I found a new lease on life and wanted to continue to the next course called Everest.

After I graduated from the Trek course, Kristina took me out to dinner. We discussed what I learned about myself, and I told her I was beyond ready to take the next step and continue on my journey to feeling better about myself.

After we returned from dinner, we did what was similar to an exit interview. Then, I signed up for the Everest course. I underwent the same process when I signed up for the Trek course. It helped me understand what I wanted from life.

That night, we went out to see a cool band. They were a cover band, and there were a lot of songs that I knew and some I didn't. It was a lot of fun. A bunch of us went out and it was great. I didn't sip alcohol, and I could still have fun.

I flew home on Tuesday and was to return to Fort Myers in about six weeks. I was so excited to return to Florida and loved everything about it. Everything was beautiful, especially the sunshine and the beach.

During the six weeks I was away from Florida, I stayed in touch with friends from Trek as often as possible and received emails from the course I took. It was good to feel involved, even though I didn't live in town. It felt like I mattered. That's all I wanted: to feel like I belonged somewhere in this world.

I still felt a little lost, but I hoped Everest would help me get through that. I felt more confident in myself and more secure in my identity.

When it was finally time to go back to Florida, I felt like I was home. The moment I got off the plane, I was where I needed to be in my life. I felt more at home than I did in Massachusetts. When Kristina picked me up, I was so excited to have more time with her and learn even more about myself.

The Everest course was different from what I expected. They started peeling the onion, as they would call it, and I cried most of the time in the course. I didn't sleep very much that weekend, but I felt even better about myself and more assertive. The whole time I was in the course, I was singing the song Stronger Woman by Jewel in my head, which came out in January of that year. There were specific lyrics that I would go over in my head. The song made me feel strong and helped me realize that no matter what happened, I would be okay.

The dark truth about the Everest course was that I was broken down and spent. I was deprived of sleep for a lot of the weekend. The first night, at ten o'clock, we were assigned a character and had to wear that costume the next day.

Before we came to class, we had to go somewhere and buy a pack of gum while wearing our costumes. The main goal was to humiliate us, even though no one would ever tell us this. They told us it would reveal to the world who we are as a person. The more you're broken down, the more likely you are to come back.

I was given Wonder Woman, meaning I wore a bra and underwear as my costume. I had to buy a pack of gum while wearing only that. I don't know how I did it. I was honestly too tired to care about what people thought of me for the 2 minutes I was in the store. I probably slept for only 2-3 hours that night.

I went into the workshop like that, and the leader was very proud of me for showing up in basically nothing. I was humiliated and not proud of myself, even though they lifted me and told me I did a great job. I was relieved to get back into regular clothes. Not everyone was dressed scantily as I was. Some people were Superman or a southern belle. Wonder Woman did suit me as a person, but my costume did not. I made a shield of some sort, but the details of that were just a blur.

On the same day, we had to do the same thing, but with less time. We were to perform a song and dress up to represent the song we were performing. We didn't have to go anywhere but to a location around 4 or 5 pm. I had to perform Express Yourself by Madonna. I don't have anything bad to say about this night at all. It was terrific and an exhilarating experience. Watching the other people perform and put their hearts and souls into it was AMAZING.

When my turn came, I wasn't expressing myself very much, so we had to stop a few times. Once I stopped caring about what other people thought, I was golden. I realized that expressing myself was key to me. The more I expressed myself, the more I felt alive. After all the performances were done, I felt on top of the world, and I truly felt at home in Florida.

The rest of the night went on, and I learned so much about myself. We were told that these things happen every time there is an Everest, and we could go to support other students. I was so in. The experience was truly exhilarating, and I couldn't wait to help other people feel the way I felt.

By the end of the night, my dopamine levels were through the roof. Everyone was not only feeling the love for each other, but some people were even starting to pair up and date. I unfortunately didn't start dating anyone. I was just happy to start feeling like myself again.

We never knew what to expect next, but we just kept going with the flow. By the end of it all, I turned into a beautiful butterfly. I had a mantra when I needed to bounce back. My mantra was: "I am a strong, beautiful, empowering woman!" When people heard me say it, they would say, "Yes, you are!" Some songs that resonated with me at the end of Everest were Express Yourself by Madonna, Butterfly by Mariah Carey, and It Feels Like Home by Chantal Kreviazuk.

By the time Sunday came, I was ready to make a HUGE change. I felt amazing and happy, and something came over me. I just wanted to live there full time. I was done with Massachusetts and my way of life there. I wasn't getting anywhere in my life. I felt stuck in a rut, and the only way to get out was to move to Fort Myers.

Kristina didn't expect to have a roommate by the end of the weekend, but my mom shipped my essentials down—clothes, medicine, and other necessities that I would need. I don't know why I didn't want to return home; I was just ready to start a new life. I was planning to stay and participate in the leadership program. I was excited, and I felt called to be a leader.

The program would cost me around $900. This was a significant amount, so Kristina and I thought of creating a fundraiser, where a food spread would be provided in exchange for donations. If I couldn't raise the money, I would have to wait, but I didn't want to - I needed that instant gratification, so I did my best to raise the necessary funds relatively quickly. Kristina and I hosted a party, where we provided a service that included food, and people could make donations by placing cash in a bowl to support my participation in the leadership program.

I was ready to embark on a new chapter in my life, to feel better about myself. I was prepared for the high of being positive all the time and being with the people I loved. I knew that this leadership program was an everyday thing and that I couldn't escape it unless I quit. But I didn't plan on quitting.

CHAPTER 7

The Program

———◇◇◇———

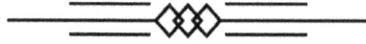

D oing leadership was an intense ride, to say the least. If you have ever worked with a life coach before, it felt like doing that every day for 90 days. You had to be on time for a coaching call; if you were late, you risked being removed from the group.

For the whole leadership course, I couldn't drink, do drugs, or have sex with anyone new. I didn't mind because I hadn't done any of the above. I was very single and just looking to focus on myself. I don't know what would happen if I broke those rules, but I didn't intend to break them.

Kristina joined leadership as a senior. Seniors were the people who had already graduated from the leadership program once. She coached students for 90 days, which was great since we could do it together. However, it was intense, and I was exhausted by the end of every day.

I was a coachee for 90 days. I knew it would be uncomfortable, but I wanted to figure out who I was and be happy. At this moment, I knew this was my purpose, no matter what I did. I deserved to have the answers, and Florida felt like the right place to find them

We had to speak with our coach at a specific time every day. We couldn't be late for our sessions; otherwise, we could be kicked out of the program if it happened more than once. I was always on time with my coaching calls.

We would go over our goals for the day. I can't remember the exact process, but we had many things to discuss. The calls would typically last about 10-15 minutes. I would call my coach, and they would be there to answer my questions.

I remember discussing who we would try to enroll in the Trek program that day. We didn't try to enroll them; we manifested that we would. This process went on for 90 days straight with no break. It was a lot to deal with. Additionally, finding a job was not my priority, which made it difficult for me to stay motivated.

Our goal was to enroll at least one person within 90 days, and ideally, it would be better if we could enroll more than one person. To keep our momentum alive, we needed to attend three leadership weekends: the first, second, and third.

For every event outside of leadership, we had to dress up because we were the pillar of the community. So, if we went to a Trek or an Everest event, we would dress up. I didn't have many dress clothes at this time in my life. I don't have them even now.

Since I didn't have a car, I took the bus every day to find a job. I grew up in a small town and always felt the need to have a car. This was my first experience taking the bus. I met some pretty interesting people while commuting. I didn't talk to many people, but the ones I did talk to were nice.

About a month after spontaneously moving to Florida, I was still looking for a job. My cousin told me to try Publix, about ten minutes down the street. Next door, there was a bus stop. It was perfect. Now, I just had to get the job.

I walked into Publix, went to the customer service desk, and asked to speak to the manager. I told the manager I was looking for a job and had just moved to Florida. We set up a meeting for a formal interview, and I was hired very quickly. He told me that I couldn't quit in 3 months. He wanted me to move up the ladder at Publix if that's what I wanted.

I told the manager I planned on staying in Florida and not moving back to Massachusetts. He knew I was taking the bus to and from work and ensured my schedule was reasonable. My cousin could pick me up if it were past when the bus was running. I think Publix closed at 10 p.m., and the bus stopped running around 9:30 p.m.

They started me as a bagger even though I wanted to be a cashier. The baggers had to bag the groceries, walk the customers out to their cars, and load them into their vehicles. It was not my favorite thing to do, but I did it. Customers would sometimes give a cash tip, which was nice. It was typically enough for a coffee, and I didn't get tipped often.

I also returned the carts to the store in 90+ degree weather. We did five carts at a time, and though they were easy to maneuver, I was not prepared for the heat or used to that kind of manual labor.

Early in my leadership, I enrolled a friend from home in the Trek program. She didn't even know that I had moved to Florida. She was ready for a change, and I was prepared to help her realize that her mindset could be transformed. I tried to enroll as many people as I could, but some people called it a cult and thought I was crazy.

I was still adamant that it wasn't a cult. Even though my whole sense of self had changed. I had a different way of speaking, and I didn't feel like I could relate to anyone who didn't talk like me.

At the end of leadership, I was ready to graduate. Before we started the festivities for the weekend, Kristina and two other friends from the program went out to check the Calusa Nature Center. It was cool to see and interact with the animals.

We went to a different nature center area, and I accidentally stepped on a fire ant hill. I wasn't wearing sneakers, and I felt like I was being stung by hundreds of bees. It was awful and it hurt and itched like nobody's business. It was one of the worst experiences I've ever had. I took some extra cortisone to make sure that I would be okay. I knew I would have to live through it for the third weekend, but I'd never itched so bad in my life.

Leadership weekend was a blast. I'm not going into details, but I loved everyone I was in leadership with. I felt incredibly free and gained a deeper perspective on who I was in this life. I felt so good about being able to complete something.

Getting through leadership gave me the permission to get through anything. I did it and I was so proud of myself. It was a long weekend, and I was exhausted by the end of it.

Since the leadership course was over, Kristina and I talked, and I decided to move back home. I was very sad about moving home, but I missed my family. My boss at Publix wasn't happy about my moving home. He told me I was ready to be a cashier, but I still decided to leave. I felt bad for only having that job for 2 months, but I was making $800 per month at that job and barely making ends meet.

I flew home, and life felt different. Everything was the same, but somehow, it wasn't. I grew significantly for 5 months, while it felt like nothing changed at home. I had changed my perspective on life and my language, and as a result, no one could understand me. I felt like I was speaking a different language, and they were talking English.

It stems from the fact that my time in Florida made me continue speaking positively. If I were honest about it, it's been 17 years since I did this program, so I don't remember what I was saying. But as an example, instead of saying "I have to", I would say "I get to".

I did end up working another job not long after I got home. I worked at a franchise doing taxes, and I thoroughly enjoyed it. I had the opportunity to meet a wide range of people. It was very chaotic for a while. We had a lot of busy days, and I was exhausted at the end of it all. I liked the hustle and bustle of the tax office. It was fun and I liked my co-workers.

In March 2009, my mom told me she was willing to do the Trek program and see what it was all about. I'm pretty sure she was suspicious that I was even more in a funk after I got home than before I left. I wasn't acting like myself at all. My mom and I weren't getting along as well as we used to. I was annoyed with her a lot more than I had been.

We flew down, and I volunteered to help over the weekend. I cried more for her breakdowns and breakthroughs than I did for my own Trek. I was so excited that my mom could finally be on the same level as me. My mom graduated, and I cried my eyes out.

I think my mom thought I was in a cult, but didn't want to say it until she took the course to experience it for herself. My mom opted not to do Everest. She just wanted to see what I had been learning and why I was acting differently. She said she got a lot out of it, but it wasn't for her. She just wanted to see what it was all about. She was trying to talk me out of the program.

My visit to Florida had a profound impact on me. I wanted to be there so bad. I felt like I was sucked back in and my only way out of feeling the pain and suffering was if I moved back to Florida.

I had some money saved up and decided I needed to find a place to live. I wasn't planning on moving back in with Kristina. I wanted to be fully on my own. I had reached out to a friend I knew who rented out apartments, and she said that she had one apartment available as of May 1st, which would cost me $1,000 a month. It was a two-bedroom duplex. I knew I couldn't afford that alone for long, so I would have to find a roommate.

I was moving to Fort Myers Beach in a little over a month. I loved the beach. It was my favorite place in the world. My apartment would be a quarter mile away from it. I felt like I was in complete serenity. The only thing was that I didn't have a car, but since it was relatively easy to get around by bus, I decided to deal with it in the meantime.

I got a flight for April 30th, and my landlord said that I could move in a day early. I packed everything I owned into two big suitcases.

I decided to rent a car for a week so I could get my bearings, find the bus stops, and find my way around Fort Myers. I knew where a lot of the places I needed to go were. I just wanted to make sure I had a vehicle to get around in.

At that time, I would've done anything to be back in Florida, where I was with "family," people who understood me. I got that high back from being back with people that I loved. And I needed to be back full-time.

I was off and on social security for quite a while at this time. I had just gotten it back, and I received some back pay for being back on it again, so I knew I would be okay for a while. I was on social security because of my medical disability. My growth hormone alone would cost $5000 per month for me to get without the extra help. I could work, but my medical condition gave me some limitations, meaning I got tired extremely fast. I did the best that I could with what life had offered me.

Panhypopituitarism is not easy by any means. At this time, one wrong move and I would go into an adrenal crisis. Forgetting my medicine was the easy part. To be honest, I don't know how I survived.

I was extremely happy to be back in Fort Myers. I found the key and brought all my stuff to the room that I chose, across from the bathroom. My place was beautiful. It was fully furnished, so I just brought myself and a ton of clothes. I unpacked and I saw a gecko out of the corner of my eye and screamed. I thought it was a mouse. I was grateful that it wasn't.

The next day, I got in touch with a friend of mine from the program. We thought it would be fun to go out and see a cover band at a cute little beach bar called The Cottage, which no longer exists due to Hurricane Ian. We went out and danced all night. I was extremely shy, so Jess, my extroverted friend, would go out and introduce me to people.

It was nice to be back in the world and to be myself again officially. I felt so lost and alone in Massachusetts. Every word that came out of my mouth felt like I was speaking gibberish.

One week after I arrived in Florida, I bought a car. It was a 2008 Chevy Cobalt. It was in a Blue Cobalt Color. It was a two-door hatchback car. I absolutely loved it. It got me around, and I was happy that I had something of my own.

In late May, I found my roommate. He was twenty-one, and he was weird. He worked on the pirate ship just off Fort Myers Beach. I wasn't home that often anyway. I just did my thing, and he pretty much did whatever he wanted. Apparently, he was on probation for something. I don't know what, since I didn't ask. My landlord was the one who found him so that I could have some help with the rent. I probably should've asked what he was on probation for.

I decided to participate in another round of leadership, and this time I would be a coach. I was thrilled to assist people with their breakdowns and help them achieve their breakthroughs.

This round of Leadership began in early June 2009, and it would be my first as a senior. At this point, I was hoping to do many rounds as a senior.

The first weekend of Leadership started, and I had a coachee with whom I was super excited. However, after a week, she decided that leadership wasn't for her. It felt like I was the one being coached, but I wasn't coaching anyone.

Another coachee dropped out, so another senior and I ended up coaching each other. Before my coaching call for the day, we'd talk to the coach above us and discuss what I should mention that day.

Everyone thought I should date the senior I was coaching. We often were pushed together, and they thought we should date. But he was ten years older, and we didn't have much in common. They just thought we were the perfect couple. No offense to him, but he wasn't my type whatsoever.

Coaching went well for a while. Then things started to change. We switched leadership for the second half, and I got another coachee. Every morning before I talked to him, I spoke to my coach, and I felt like I would get yelled at every day.

I don't know what I was doing wrong, but I was pushed to tell my coachee things because he wasn't achieving his goals or enrolling people.

My success mirrored his success, and vice versa. According to them, I wasn't doing my job, and they weren't happy with me.

I was so depressed and sad all the time. I remember telling my mom that I was having a hard time, and she told me that I could get out of it any time. I told her I know, but I just don't know what to do with my life.

The only thing that made me happy at the end of the day was going out to see the cover band with friends. I would go as much as possible. They would either be down the street at the cottage or 15 minutes away. It was nice to make friends with people. That one band gave me a better community than I had in the program. I wasn't drinking; going out and dancing with friends was just fun.

I was nicknamed Dancing Nancy. It's kind of a name I gave myself, but it stuck since it suited me. Dancing Nancy is a Dave Matthews Band song that I loved. I believe it was on my Facebook or Myspace at the time, and it just became my name.

Leadership ended, and I was beyond relieved. I was so happy to be able to move on. I stayed with the program for about two more months. I waited until I moved out to leave. I remember attending an event with a friend and saying I was done. I never went back.

I would see people here and there, but I realized that I had lost myself as a person. I wanted to be myself again. I wanted to be happy and healthy. I tried to speak like I did before I joined a self-help program that turned into a cult. Okay, maybe it wasn't a full-fledged cult, but it had the potential to get there. The more people who were enrolled, the more it brought people together. If you look at Steven Hassan's Bite Model, a lot of things in the model were in this program.

I was proud of myself for leaving. I wanted to get back to being myself. I felt like I lost a massive part of who I was. I felt like I was holding a secret that I could tell no one. We weren't allowed to tell anyone about the program. No details whatsoever. The program I was in utilized NLP, or neuro-linguistic programming, to change our behaviors and the world around us.

Neuro-linguistic programming is a set of techniques that utilize language to help individuals modify their thoughts and behaviors. So what I was going through was real. Every time I left for a weekend, I was super pumped and ready to go. I would speak differently and I would act differently. It was like I was being brainwashed, even though they promised that's not what they were doing.

I made a very close friend from the group, and we stayed friends after I left. Jo became my best friend, and when I moved to Cape Coral, we lived five minutes from each other, which made life easy. She was an extrovert, and we formed many good friendships. We went to Key West and stayed out with friends until 4 a.m. My friend group expanded a lot after that weekend.

We had such a fun time together. I did make new friends from Key West, and we went out together a lot. It was fun to have friends to go out with every week. That one little group of people became my friends for life. We may not all talk often, but they all mean the world to me to this day.

In early March, on a Wednesday, I went out with some friends I met in Key West. I was excited because I didn't have to drive. I loved watching those guys sing and do their job. This was a small bar in Cape Coral, and I loved it a lot. It's still one of my favorite places to this day, though I haven't been there in about 6 years.

I talked to my mom before I went out, and I said that I was excited to have fun. I also spoke with my best friend, Rae. They both said I sounded like I was in good spirits.

We had a blast dancing and having a great time. I got a little drunk. I wasn't driving, so I didn't have to worry much about it.

I don't remember any part of that night. I don't even remember going out. Not because I was blacked out drunk, but because I stopped taking my medication. I was very skinny. I wasn't taking care of myself.

On Friday, my cousin Kristina noticed that I wasn't on Facebook and became worried about me. I was always on Facebook. She tried calling me, and I wouldn't answer the phone. She headed over to where I was living and found me on the floor. I was very close to death.

All I remember was waking up in the hospital, and my mom being there. I was sedated for a day or two. I was hooked up to a ventilator, so my throat hurt a lot.

The doctors were worried that I had brain damage because I was doing a stretching motion. My mom knew it was normal, since I always stretch my arms over my head when I wake up in the morning. She just said, "That's Nancy's way of waking up."

All my tests came back normal, and the doctor was going to release me to a normal floor, but my mom said that I needed to be released from the hospital. If I were okay with leaving the ICU, I would be fine with returning to Massachusetts. She didn't want me to catch anything else while I was there. I barely remember being in the hospital or what happened to me.

That was the worst adrenal crisis I had ever had. Even though it was self-induced because I believed I didn't need my medication. Waking up in the hospital on a ventilator gave me a wake-up call, and I vowed to be better at taking my medication and taking care of myself.

I went home. Everyone was relieved I would be okay and get the help I needed. I was happier being home. I could see my family and friends, and that's all that mattered. That doesn't mean I didn't miss the beautiful Florida weather, though.

I got home and went to see my endocrinologist the very next day. I was in pretty good shape, except for being weak. My endocrinologist said, "I never expected to see you again." Right then, I knew it was time to change doctors. I believe I saw him for a year or more, until I found an endocrinologist who suited me better.

I spent my 30th birthday with my best friend, Rae. We went to a local bar and had a great time with her family. I just needed my best friend and was happy to be with her.

Coming home was different from what I expected. I was happy to be home, and even though life didn't go as I wanted, it was the right choice for me. I missed Florida a lot, but my mom said there was no reason that I couldn't visit.

One thing about going back home that bothered me was rumors spreading about why I ended up in the hospital. Some people were saying that it was because I went out drinking.

The truth is, I ended up in the hospital because I stopped taking care of myself. I stopped taking my medication. I wanted to be normal and not worry about having panhypopituitarism. I wanted to go out and have fun without thinking about taking my next dose.

Being normal was the whole goal at this point in my life. I wanted to be able to spontaneously go away for a weekend. I didn't want to constantly have my medication on my mind. But I couldn't do that because, if I did, I wouldn't be here writing this book.

When you live with a rare disease, you feel isolated since no one besides your mother can understand it. No one knows why I'm feeling groggy or slurring my words—the two main symptoms for me of an adrenal crisis.

When there's no community to fall back on, it's hard to cope. It feels like no one can relate to you, especially when you don't want to take your medication or when you don't understand why you still need to take it at thirty.

Luckily, in 2025, I no longer have that problem as long as I take my medication once a day. I can be normal. It's taken me a long time to get to where I am today. I couldn't have done it without my endocrinologist.

Once I take my medication, I can go all day without having to worry. All I need aside from it is my growth hormone, which I take at night. It's something I will need for at least the next 20 years, if I'm lucky, and for the rest of my life.

Living with Panhypopituitarism has given me the strength to become who I am today. At this point in my life, I don't know who I would be without this rare disease. If it weren't for the challenges I faced, some of which I had created on my own, I wouldn't be the person I am today.

While the program I was in had some cult-like qualities, it played a significant role in shaping me. I'm forever grateful for that. Without them, I wouldn't have met the amazing people I know today. I don't believe I would have any interest in the self-help industry if I didn't have that program. It helped me learn that it was okay to want more for myself.

CHAPTER 8

What I Didn't Know

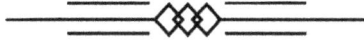

N ot long after I moved home from Florida, my mom and I talked. I told her that I didn't understand panhypopituitarism. I knew I had it, but I didn't understand the extent of it.

I knew my pituitary gland didn't function, that it was torn off and floating on the other side of my brain. I knew that I took medications because of it. But why? How do these medications help me? Why do I take them?

I was clueless, and I sadly had no idea why my medicine was important. I felt uneducated about my rare disease. I had been living for thirty years at this point. You would think I would know more about panhypopituitarism. Maybe I would be more responsible if I knew what my medication did to make my life easier.

Having panhypopituitarism in 2010, there were barely any resources. I couldn't just Google when I should increase my steroids and have an answer pop up. I had to dig deep and figure it out on my own.

I did searches for panhypopituitarism, and barely anything came up. If it did, it wasn't someone that I could talk to. It was a foundation that focused on children with panhypopituitarism.

I was desperate to know someone who had panhypopituitarism just to realize I wasn't alone. So I came up with an idea. I heard that Facebook had a business page feature, so I started a Facebook business page called

Panhypopituitarism. I would update it periodically, adding motivational quotes to motivate people on their journey. It wasn't a place to have a conversation. It was a place to show other patients I was ready to figure this out.

I used Facebook Ads, and it helped me get started to find new followers. By the time I had 100 followers, I felt like I was doing okay. I felt like I belonged somewhere, but I was still searching for a female who was born with panhypopituitarism around my age.

I didn't feel alone anymore. I had no idea if I would ever do anything with that Facebook page, but it helped me realize that it wasn't just me who dealt with this condition. At this point, that's all I needed—proof—proof that I wasn't alone, and I was just happy to have that. Before I deleted that Facebook page, I had over 650 followers and I was proud that I was making a little progress in life.

In August 2011, I started a part-time job at JCPenney in the shoe department. I worked extremely hard. I had to climb ladders and find shoes for people of all sizes. We got a commission, but it wasn't much.

I slowly got into the swing of things. I liked it, and the other employees liked me as well. It was great, overall. My job was a mix of sales, assisting customers with shoe try-ons, and everything in between. It was a lot of running around, though, and my feet didn't love me for it.

On September 3, 2011, I had the morning off because I was going to the Apple Store in New Hampshire. We didn't have one nearby, so I drove 90 minutes just to pick up my iPhone 4s. I was thrilled; I love Apple and all its products.

On my way to work around 3 p.m., I stopped by Grace's house to see my niece and nephew and show them my new iPhone! I was so happy. I've always been a tech nerd. I loved anything related to technology.

Grace had her birthday the day before, and we were chatting when the phone suddenly rang. I knew it was Dad on the phone because she mentioned it was him before she picked up.

Grace figured Dad was calling to wish her a Happy Belated Birthday. He didn't call her yesterday, and it was unusual for him not to call on our birthdays. Even when we don't talk to him often, he still called to wish us a Happy Birthday.

I knew something was wrong by the look on her face, and she started crying. Grace handed me the phone, and Dad told me that he didn't have much longer to live. He had stage 4 lung cancer, and he was dying. He said it would take a few weeks to a month, if lucky. Chemo wasn't an option at this point. We would just have to wait and see.

Grace and I drove to our Mom's house and waited for her to get home before we called anyone else. As far as we could tell, we were the first to find out. Our only choice was to fly to Las Vegas and be with our Dad. We would be there as much as we could until he passed.

We cried it out together, called our family members, and told them to meet at our aunt's house. The next day, we all planned to fly to Las Vegas.

My dad's side of the family flew to Las Vegas 24 hours later, and I was scared and anxious. I didn't know what to think. We had seen our dad just a few months ago. He looked fine.

This year was the most we'd ever seen him. He was a long-distance truck driver. He was laid off from his job and didn't tell us about this change until he was just about ready to graduate from school. It was a job that he wanted, he said, for a long time. He wanted to drive across the country.

When we arrived in Las Vegas, it was such a hard time for all of us, and a majority of it was spent crying and hugging each other. Dad didn't look good, and I was scared of spending time with him. I didn't want to cry in front of him, but it was too hard not to. I didn't want to say goodbye.

My dad wasn't the perfect father figure. We weren't the closest, but he was still my dad. When I was younger, I made sure I stayed in touch. I didn't want him to forget I existed because life moved on whether we wanted it to or not. We spent as much time with him and his wife, Carol. My dad meant a lot to me, even though he wasn't always there for us.

My job was not supportive of my having to travel back, even though my dad was dying. I had been there for about a month. They told me to make a choice: either quit or come back to work and not be with my family. The obvious choice was to be with my dad, so I quit. They told me I could come back when I was ready; all I had to do was reapply. I was not willing to do that. I was upset that I couldn't just take a short leave of absence. Losing a parent is not easy for anyone, especially when they live on the other side of the country.

We all went home for about a week to attend to a few things that required our attention. Even with Dad's diagnosis, life has an ironic way of moving forward. We returned to Las Vegas afterwards. We knew it was the last time that we would see Dad alive, and it hurt a lot. In less than 24 hours of us getting there, he went to the hospice center because he was jaundiced. They were going to keep him comfortable until he passed, and we knew it was the end.

Watching my dad deteriorate in front of my eyes is the hardest thing that I have ever experienced. In just a week, he got progressively worse. I didn't want him to see me cry, but there were just times when I couldn't help it.

The last time Dad said anything, he said, "The truck is slowing down," meaning his rig. We knew his life flashed before his eyes, and it was time to say goodbye. We left his room around 9 p.m. and went back to our hotel room to get some rest.

We were in Las Vegas when Dad died. It was around 2 a.m., and Grace's phone rang. Carol said Dad didn't have much longer, and she was heading to the hospice to be by his side. We should head there as soon as possible to say our goodbyes.

We got up and got ready to head to the hospice center. I remember this moment as if it were yesterday. I was in the bathroom, getting my clothes out of the closet. Something told me to look up, and I remember saying, "Bye, Daddy," like I was talking to him on the phone. I knew he was gone, and his spirit came to say goodbye to me.

Less than two minutes later, we received the call that he had passed. The nurse said she left the room momentarily, and when she returned, he was gone. My dad was a private person who wanted to die alone. He didn't want anyone to suffer.

Seeing his body there just made it so hard to let go. We were waiting for him to wake up and tell us that he loved us. Our dad being gone forever just hurt a lot. It still hurts 14 years later that he missed out on the amazing parts of our lives. I believe if he were here today, he'd be proud of us.

Within 17 days of getting the call, we lost our dad to stage four lung cancer. He passed away on September 20th, 2011.

He found out two weeks before and was having difficulty telling us. I believe he found out sooner and just didn't tell anyone. He wanted to travel and live out his last year to the best of his ability, spending time with his daughters and talking to them as much as possible. When I wasn't in Las Vegas, I spoke to him on the phone every day. Each day, his voice got weaker, making it so hard not to be with him.

After he passed, we packed up as much of his stuff as possible and shipped it back to Grace's house. Everything he had was ours. He didn't have many possessions, and we didn't take any furniture.

My Dad had been a smoker since he was in his teens. We knew his death would be inevitable, but we didn't think it would happen so soon. Moving on without him was unimaginable at that time. There were days I just wanted to call him and hear his voice, but I couldn't anymore.

Dad was cremated and Carol brought his ashes to Massachusetts to bury him with our grandparents. We had a small service for him and then a reception at a local rod and gun club.

There are many days when I wish he were still here, but I believe that everything happens for a reason. It was my dad's time to go.

I still think of him often. I imagine that today, he would be so proud of me for writing this book because he knew I was a creative writer. Just before he died, he gave me one of his cameras, which I kept until a couple of years ago when I gave it to my nephew. It wasn't for me to use; it was for me to pass it along to the next generation.

Not long after we lost my dad, I got a full-time job at a call center. I did six weeks of training and I loved it. It was great to have a job. In that training period, I had a lot of fun and made friends pretty easily. I believe it helped my grieving process. My first shift was 12 p.m. to 9 p.m. It was a lot of fun working late hours. Typically, after 8 p.m., it would slow down a little bit. I was ready to get out of there by 9 p.m.

Sometime in 2012, I went to my first endocrinologist appointment on my own. It was time for me to fully take care of myself and my medications. I searched around and saw a couple of different endocrinologists before reaching out to my pediatric endocrinologist and asking for a referral to one in Boston. She referred me to the Neuroendocrine department at Massachusetts General Hospital.

I recall meeting my current endocrinologist and providing him with my paperwork, as well as any relevant information about myself that I could. He got me all set up. We conducted a cortisol stimulation test to determine if I had any cortisol in my system. We did an MRI of my brain, and I got genetic testing done as well. He made sure he knew everything he could about me and my medical condition so he knew how best to treat me.

For those of you curious about the genetic testing, my panhypopituitarism was completely environmental. There was no indication that it was a genetic mutation whatsoever. If something comes up, they will notify me in the future. He was the first endocrinologist that I had seen who did a full array of tests from the first visit.

At that point, I learned a lot from my endocrinologist. He helped me understand why I needed my medication. I told him that I had no idea why I had been taking this medication for most of my life. Not only did I feel listened to by my doctor, but I also felt educated. After all, they're there to help us understand our condition.

The whole neuroendocrine team at the Massachusetts General Hospital is amazing. If you're someone in Massachusetts with an endocrine issue, I highly recommend them.

I had my last day of work at the call center in June 2013. I only lasted there about 18 months, and I was okay with that. As time passed, the call center grew increasingly loud, making it difficult for us to understand the customers. It wasn't the job for me anymore.

I took some time off to find what I wanted to do next. I spent moments decompressing and enjoying life. I devoted a lot of time to my niece and nephew, as well as Rae and her son. It was great to enjoy life.

One day in August 2013, I was watching TV in my bedroom when Andy came in and asked me why I used closed captioning on my TV. I said, "It's because I live below you and don't want the volume too loud." Then he said, "Can you hear OK?"

I didn't know how to answer that question. I thought I could hear fine—I've been hearing the same way my whole life. Both Mom and Andy encouraged me to go for a hearing test. I made an appointment with an audiologist that Andy had previously visited, and I scheduled a hearing test.

Two weeks later, I went to get my first hearing test since I was in elementary school, and I found out that I was hearing impaired with something called otosclerosis. It's an easy fix and surgery, but never in my 33 years did I think I was hearing impaired.

I'm not sure if I remember the percentages correctly, but my right side had 65% hearing loss while my left side had 45% hearing loss. Though at my last audiologist appointment, the percentages are now the same.

I have what is called conductive hearing loss. This means that the sound coming from the outside of the ear never reaches the middle ear. It's like trying to hear with earplugs on. For the first time, I found out that I was hearing impaired, and I didn't know what to think.

My audiologist referred me to an ENT (ears, nose, and throat) specialist in Worcester, MA. Mom and I met with him, and he said he was sure it was Otosclerosis, a common cause of middle-ear hearing loss. We could consider surgery, and I would be able to hear without any issues, according to his expert opinion.

Mom and I went to Tufts in Boston for what was supposed to be a 45-minute surgery. They would first operate on my right ear. My left ear would be dealt with later on. After 1 hour and 30 minutes, my mom knew something wasn't right. When the ENT came out of surgery (2 whole hours after we got to the medical center) to talk to my mom, the surgeon said my ear was nowhere near what he anticipated. It was not otosclerosis; it was something much more complicated, and he wasn't willing to explore any ways to fix my hearing. He said what I really had couldn't be fixed.

We did an MRI, and something definitely was wrong, but we'll get into that later. He said he put a prosthesis in my right ear, and we left it at that. I didn't know what that was, and at this point, I still don't know what it means. According to my research on Google, it's a piece of removable plastic that helps the ear maintain its normal shape.

After surgery, I got an MRI done to check my left ear and to make sure that it wasn't the same on the other side. Unfortunately, it was.

I asked the specialist if there was anything else he could do to help me hear normally, and he said that I could get in-ear hearing aids. In-ear hearing aids were a horrible choice, since my inner ears don't work whatsoever. Yes, it helped amplify what I was hearing, but it didn't have a significant impact on me.

I had heard about an option called a bone-anchored hearing aid since I had conductive hearing loss. They were meant for my type of hearing. A bone-anchored hearing aid goes behind the ear and is attached to the skull. When I mentioned it to the specialist, he said that he wasn't willing to help me with it, that I could only do regular hearing aids because they wouldn't work. He didn't want to explore other options or even conduct another surgery, so I dealt with in-the-ear hearing aids. I never saw him again after that.

Now, I didn't *just* have panhypopituitarism. I had panhypopituitarism, and was hearing impaired on top of that. We'll get more into my hearing impairment in the next chapter.

Not long after my unnecessary surgery, my mom found a Facebook group called PanHypoPituitarism. We were both thrilled at the thought of FINALLY meeting people with panhypopituitarism. I felt less lost, thinking I had finally found people I could relate to. I made some good friends and was ready to find my panhypopituitarism tribe.

But there was a slight problem with this group. There weren't just people who were born without a functioning pituitary gland; some of the members were also those who had pituitary tumors. It felt like a gut punch knowing there was more than one version of panhypopituitarism.

Things in the group went well, though. I met many new people and learned about pituitary tumors. Things started to get confusing because I didn't know if people were talking about whether they had a pituitary tumor or congenital panhypopituitarism.

You may wonder why the difference between the two is so confusing. I have congenital panhypopituitarism, which means I never created a single hormone on my own. Like I said, my pituitary gland is floating around the other side of my brain. It doesn't work whatsoever.

There are two types of pituitary tumors: microadenomas and macroadenomas. Microadenomas are small, while macroadenomas are bigger. Most are benign and non-cancerous, but they can cause other problems, such as vision issues and headaches.

There are cancerous pituitary tumors, too, but they're rarer, and they move on to other parts of the body. An adenoma just stays in the pituitary region. According to my research, adenomas can be removed if they cause issues or press against something that can affect quality of life. Regardless of their size, I believe they should be removed. However, many endocrinologists don't think that the tumor should be removed because it doesn't affect the overall quality of life.

Most adenomas can increase hormones, such as growth hormone, which can cause acromegaly or gigantism, which can cause one to grow too fast. They also have prolactinoma, which can cause your body to feel like it's pregnant, and have breast milk and hormonal acne. There's also Cushing's disease, which means they make too much cortisol. The list goes on and on.

It becomes hypopituitarism or panhypopituitarism after surgery or after radiation treatments. When one or more of the hormones stop working, some people need all of the hormones replaced, and some don't.

This side of panhypopituitarism became more confusing than it was, making it hard to understand everything at once. It's just several facts thrown at you at the same time, and you don't know which side of the spectrum is what. It's hard to piece things together sometimes.

Even so, finding this group was life-changing for me. This was my first taste of what it felt like to be understood in this world. Before the internet, as a kid growing up with a rare disease, it was incredibly difficult to find someone with a similar condition. Finding people with a similar rare disease is easier nowadays, thanks to things like Facebook groups.

I spent as much time as possible in this group and tried to find my tribe—people identical to me. It wasn't hard, but it wasn't easy either.

After I got my first set of hearing aids in 2014, I decided it was time to get a part-time job, just to get out of the house and be more social. I didn't want to be sitting in my parents' basement all day. Luckily, I found a part-time job at a testing center. I worked about 16-30 hours, and every once in a while, I would work 40 hours.

This testing center provided tests of all types for doctors, dentists, insurance professionals, accountants, and others. I started this job in 2014. I liked it for the most part. Things did get boring after everyone had gone in to take their tests.

We would have to go in every 10 minutes and walk around the room to make sure that no one was cheating. Every test taker's breaks were different. Some could go into their lockers and some couldn't. Some had 8-hour tests, while others had a 4-hour test. There was a lot to keep track of, but I felt better having a job to focus on. Other aspects of my life were getting better, too.

In May 2015, I was tired of getting confused about who had what kind of panhypopituitarism, which was called PHP for short and CPHP if you have congenital panhypopituitarism. So, I decided to create a group called Congenital Panhypopituitarism. This group was for people who were born with panhypopituitarism and were diagnosed without a functioning pituitary gland later in life. In 2025, we have over 700 members, and this group will celebrate its 10th anniversary in May. I can't believe how fast time has gone by.

This group is a dream come true. I loved talking to people and learning about their experiences with panhypopituitarism. We answered questions and talked about our experiences with panhypopituitarism.

We're not doctors, but as a community, we have gained extensive experience that enables us to help each other as best as possible. We all have our own experiences, so I made a specific rule in the group that states there are no wrong answers.

Living with panhypopituitarism is an experience in itself, with each day feeling completely different from another. One day, we're up and ready to go; the next, we're in bed, not feeling well. Every day brings new challenges, but as long as we take care of ourselves and take our medication on time, we won't have much of an issue.

There are days when I feel utterly exhausted, but I keep pushing through. Learning what I have up until this point about my medication and myself has helped me a great deal. I feel like I finally belong, and I am no longer isolated.

It felt like a weight lifted off my shoulders, and I could finally be in a community where living with panhypopituitarism was normal. They may not be a part of my everyday life, but they helped me cope and learn a great deal from each other.

CHAPTER 9

Leashes, Lessons, and Learning to Lead

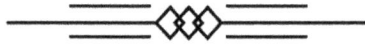

━━━━◇◆◇━━━━

T hings were starting to go well. I gained a lot of confidence, especially when it came to my group. The members were teaching me more than I was teaching them.

Our group is set up rather simply. People ask questions, and other members (including me) answer as best as we can. In our group, everyone has their own experiences, so I let the members know there were no wrong answers. There's a reason why I did that. If you join other groups, you can see a lot of arguments and members disagreeing with each other. I didn't want our group to become like that, and thanks to my rule, it didn't.

At the start of the summer of 2016, I was let go from my job at the testing center, along with a few others. I was okay with it since I was already looking for something new. The testing center was becoming stricter with its policies and was getting more challenging. New cameras were installed, monitoring our every move. We had to scan people with a metal detector. I was not up to their standards in that regard. I was pretty bored at my job - it felt like the days dragged on.

After I got home from losing my job, my mom and I were talking. I was on Pinterest, of all places, looking for simple work-from-home jobs or freelance jobs. I came upon something called Rover. Rover was for people who wanted to be a dog walker or pet sitter but didn't want to start a business. It was more for those who wanted to do dog walking as a side gig.

I was okay with being on Rover part-time until I found another job. So, I signed up for it. I loved it. I loved working with animals. It was so much fun, and the money wasn't bad. I figured I would do it for the rest of the summer and see what happened. I ended up with 5-star reviews, and I was over the moon and passionate about what I was doing.

I was always busy, and I decided that it could be a thriving business. I went from being bored at a job that I didn't love to playing with animals all day. Nothing was better at this point in my life. I felt like I was on top of the world, and I finally felt like I was ready for something new. I felt like at 36, I could do this for the rest of my life.

I loved taking care of animals. I felt delighted that I got to take care of cats and dogs. I decided to launch my own pet sitting business called Nancy's Pet Sitting. My launch date was January 1, 2017, and I was excited to finally start doing something on my own, without having to worry about signing in and out.

I was my own boss. I was thrilled to be a new business owner. I loved building a business from scratch. There wasn't much out there in 2017. You had to learn from Facebook Groups or Pet Sitters International.

There are only a few things needed when you're starting a pet sitting business: a license from your town/city and pet sitters' insurance. That's all I had at that time. I didn't have any software or similar tools. I conducted my business with pen and paper, which made things quite challenging at times, especially when it comes to scheduling. Google Calendar was my best friend when it came to scheduling, and it still is to this day.

I posted for the first time in the town's local Facebook group, and I started to get clients pretty quickly. My business took off like a rocket, thriving more than I had hoped. I met amazing clients who liked me. I was traveling within a 15-mile radius of my house in Hubbardston and was thrilled to be doing so well. I didn't need Rover anymore, and that was a good thing. By the summer of 2017, I was consistently booked, and I loved every second of it.

Pet sitting gave me so many opportunities. I wasn't just working with cats and dogs. I was working with alpacas, chickens, donkeys, rabbits, and more. It was just the best thing ever. I loved my job. Most days, I worked from 9 a.m. to 3 p.m., but I also enjoyed many vacation pet-sits. I would start my day at 6 a.m. and end at 9 p.m. It was a long shift, but I took many breaks and I thoroughly enjoyed what I did.

Pet sitting allowed me to return to Fort Myers, see friends, and party like I wasn't in my late 30s. I saw friends I met after the program, and was beyond happy to have them back in my life. I began taking better care of myself. I took my medication consistently, and I rarely ever missed a dose. During the times I accidentally missed or forgot one, I was immediately exhausted. I couldn't win no matter what I did regarding fatigue.

My medication was making it increasingly difficult to run my business. I had to take my hydrocortisone dose three times a day. Hydrocortisone, as a steroid, is metabolized in the body within 8 hours. When the medicine wore off after those 8 hours, I was completely drained. I had to use alarms to remind myself to take my next dose.

I describe being on hydrocortisone as running out of gas. When your car runs out of gas, you need to fill it back up to get back on the road. Hydrocortisone is very similar to this scenario. The medication would only work for a selected period, and then my body would force me to fall asleep. I could stay awake if I were driving, obviously, but my energy would only last me so long.

Running an active business with this rare disease makes things complicated. I always had to make sure I kept my hydrocortisone in my car or on my person at all times, and I had alarms set to make sure I took my medication at the correct times. Otherwise, I was not going to make it through the day. I would try to time it around 7 hours to make sure that I get my medication on time.

But I loved every facet of my business. Although I didn't have any pets at the time, I loved spending time with animals. I was always the girl at the party playing with animals rather than talking to people. That's me to this day.

I met another pet sitter in my area who became my mentor, and I assisted her as my skills grew. When you're trying to run and grow your business, it's not easy to freelance at the same time. Sometimes it's just one or the other. I stayed with her for about a year until I got too busy to help her full-time. I helped as much as I could, though.

As I onboarded new clients, I became increasingly busy. It was challenging, but I became very good at scheduling myself down to the minute. It was a puzzle, but it was something that I loved to do. I didn't have any software at the time. I mostly handled cash and checks, so I became an expert at managing my business on my own. I felt entirely in the groove.

There is a downfall in the pet sitting industry, though. Burnout is a considerable facet, especially when you don't have employees. I probably could've hired someone by the beginning of 2018, but I didn't want to grow that big. I didn't want to be anyone's boss.

I remember working 16 hours on a particularly long day. I left my house at 6 a.m. and didn't get home until 10 p.m. I had to stop at the local pizza place to pick up a pizza for dinner because it was well after 6 p.m., and I was starving. I ate it on the way to my next client. Trust me, it was only one day; I never stretched myself that thin again.

I had four clients at a time, and all of them were pet-sitting clients. If you don't know what pet sitting is, it involves 3 to 4 visits per day, with each visit lasting approximately half an hour. This wasn't a lot of time for the dogs to be outside, but it was the industry standard, and most dogs were okay with it. Unfortunately, not all dogs adapted to the pet-sitting schedule. There were hard days when I would walk into houses to potty accidents that no one wanted to come home to. I made sure any accidents were cleaned up before I left, which is a lot of work for a half-hour visit. I was always happy at the end of every summer because it meant my busy season was over and I could return to my regular schedule.

In 2018, my mom drove me to my endocrinologist in Boston. It was during a bad storm, and I felt sick. I had a cold that wouldn't go away for 3 weeks. My mom told me to triple my dose so I would feel okay.

Driving to Boston was fine. We didn't experience any major issues getting there with the snow. This was the first time my mom had accompanied me to my endocrinologist in over six years.

When I walked in, I warned him that I had a cold and I wasn't feeling great. I told him that I had been stress-dosing my hydrocortisone to help get over this illness. He asked me why. I told him that it's what I've always done in the past. I was taught to increase my dose when I had a cold or wasn't feeling well.

My neuroendocrinologist taught me a crucial lesson that day. I should only increase if I have a fever, a broken bone, or surgery. Otherwise, I should take my regular dose. After that visit, I followed his instructions, and I was better within 48 hours of taking my regular dose. I've only had one fever and three surgeries since 2018.

That day, I stopped increasing my dose for every little thing that stressed me out. I used to increase every time I was stressed out or had a busy day because that's what my endocrinologists and other doctors taught me, but just because I *felt* stressed didn't mean my body was. What I realized was that increasing my dose when I was sick brought my immune system down, making me sicker. I would go from having a cold to bronchitis because I increased my dose for so long that it didn't give my body enough time to recuperate. When I finally stopped, my illness went away almost immediately.

What I've noticed since I've been off my increased doses is that I hardly ever get sick. I would maybe have one cold per year, otherwise I'm healthy as a horse. I've learned that an increased dose makes me extremely tired. Like I can hardly stand, never mind be awake enough to eat. It takes me at least two to three days to get back to my usual self, especially after surgery.

Within a year after that conversation, I learned the rules for increasing my hydrocortisone. I started to feel like a normal person once I realized that it wasn't necessary to increase my dose. I decided to make a change and talked to my endocrinologist about getting on prednisone as an option. Most of his patients were on prednisone, and it was a once-a-day solution. He said I could try it.

I went from taking medication thrice per day to once a day, and it's been a fantastic change for me. Going on prednisone permitted me to be normal. It allowed me to understand that I could live with my rare disease and still thrive daily.

You may be thinking, you were on this before, and it didn't work, so why does it work now? The last time I was on it, I was on the wrong dose. I believe I was on 5 mg when I should've been on 3mg.

I can wake up and get on with my day, rather than spending multiple hours in bed. I rarely take naps anymore, and it's because my body is stable throughout the day. I don't have to worry about going into an adrenal crisis.

I do want to address why I don't increase my medication before I move forward. Stress dosing is a very controversial topic within the panhypopituitarism community. If you or someone you know has panhypopituitarism, you may be yelling at this book right now.

Increasing my dose would sometimes have the opposite effect, and I would stay up all night until 5 or 6 a.m. Doing it while sick made my body take much longer to recover. If my body isn't under stress, I feel fine - I rarely ever have a problem. I haven't had an adrenal crisis in 15 years, and I'm proud of myself for that.

Taking too many steroids can give our bodies many issues. One issue is moon face. If you didn't know, it's when you have too much cortisol in your system, and your face starts to swell. Too many steroids can also give you non-alcoholic fatty liver disease.

Always check with your endocrinologist about anything related to your cortisol levels. Remember, I am talking as a patient; this is my way of doing things that suits my life. I am not an endocrinologist. I'm just relaying what I've been taught.

In 2019, I decided to get a second opinion about my hearing. I met with an otologist who was very informative about the current state of my hearing loss. She's at Mass Eye and Ear, and she only focuses on ears. She's a phenomenal doctor.

Before I saw her, I did an MRI of my head so she could see what the inner part of my ears looked like. When she saw them, she said they didn't look good. She said that my inner ear was blocked by bone, and she helped me come up with better options to improve my hearing.

My hearing loss is hard to explain. The easiest way to put it is that bone blocks my inner ear, making my normal ears nonfunctional. The best way to describe my hearing loss is to imagine grabbing two earplugs that block sound, getting a sewing needle, and putting one hole in each from top to bottom. Put the earplugs in and try to hear normally. That's how I hear when I don't wear my cochlear implant. I hear okay when I use the hearing aid feature with my AirPod Pros, but it's not nearly as good as my cochlear hearing aids.

The doctor was surprised I could hear at all. She told me it's like listening through a pinhole. They could not do surgery on my actual ear because there is no way to get the bone out of it. So, I opted for something else.

With conductive hearing loss, there are options that the other doctor wasn't willing to explore. There is a type of hearing aid called bone-anchored hearing aids, which conduct sound through the mastoid bone.

I opted for the surgery. My first surgery was in my right ear for the BAHA 5 Attract. This means a magnet is implanted in my mastoid bone and is attached to a magnet on the other side of my skin.

The surgery wasn't that bad, but the entire process took a remarkably long time - approximately 4-5 hours. The one thing I needed for the surgery was extra hydrocortisone. I get 100 mg of hydrocortisone for any surgery I have.

After my first surgery, my doctor said something else that was very surprising to me. The reason for my clumsiness was that I didn't have a vestibular system since my inner ear was full of bone. I couldn't ride a bike or a motorcycle even if I wanted to. My mom was shocked when she heard the news. We also laughed. My family had tried to get me to ride a bike for hours when I was younger. People also said they'd teach me, but I never got too far, even after my body got used to balancing. I would do great for a second, and then I would fall. I was able to ride a bike briefly in the past (as mentioned in the previous chapters). Those few seconds felt freeing. It was great, but I don't want to relive them. I'm okay standing on my own two feet.

That doesn't mean I can do so without injuring myself, though. I've probably fallen at least a few hundred times over the last forty-five years of my life. I'm so glad that with all those falls, I only broke one bone. I always have one bad fall a year. Most of the time, when I fall, I always land on my knees. I never would've thought my balance issues were related to my ears.

For after-surgery care, I couldn't bend or lift more than 5 lbs for 2 weeks. By the following Tuesday, I was okay to go back to dog walking. I had no problems related to the surgery, but I was required to wear a cone over the area where the surgery was done. The easiest way to describe it is as a curved oval shape, and gauze was wrapped around my head to hold it in place. I had to keep it that way for 48 hours before washing my hair.

It was awful to sleep in, but the pain wasn't that bad. They gave me pain meds, but I didn't take them and just used extra-strength Tylenol. I was also on antibiotics for a while.

If there was anything about my surgery that was hard, I would say it would be coming out of the anesthesia and weaning off the 100 mg of hydrocortisone. I remember throwing up after my first surgery, which isn't unusual. Plus, they drilled a hole into my skull. I could not hold anything down without projectile vomiting. Luckily, I didn't get sick after that.

Six weeks after surgery, I got my BAHA Attract device for my right ear. I was so happy I could finally hear more than the muffled sounds I was accustomed to with my normal hearing.

This device opened up a whole new world, and I loved every second of it. I went from barely hearing anything to hearing just about everything. I wouldn't say I had a 100% hearing, but it was definitely somewhere around 90%.

The only issue I had with my hearing aid was that it would screech a lot. It got annoying. I couldn't nap with it on or put my hair up without hearing a bit of screeching. So, I wore my hair down and lived with it until there was a better solution.

My otologist wanted to see me 6 months after the surgery. I told her that I wanted to get a bone-anchored hearing aid for my left ear. This occurred in late 2019, before the COVID-19 pandemic. She told me that they were introducing a device called the Osia 2, and that I would be the perfect candidate for it. We scheduled my surgery for mid-February 2020, just before everything started to shut down. I was so happy that I would be able to hear out of both of my ears for my 40th birthday. That was always the goal, especially when I had the option of getting hearing aids that would work for me.

When the fear of COVID-19 hit, I was hoping that the United States wouldn't end up in a pandemic. I had never lived through one before, and I wasn't too happy that it might happen at this point in life.

By mid-March, things started to shut down rather quickly, and I was so upset when they cancelled my activation appointment. I wouldn't be able to get my second implant to be able to hear on my 40th birthday.

I spoke with my otologist, and she was able to schedule an appointment for me. The worst place to be at the start of COVID was a hospital or a place with sick people. Luckily for me, I was in Mass Eye and Ear. I got in and out as fast as I possibly could.

Mass Eye and Ear has mostly valet-only parking, and the valet was shut down, so I had to find parking by myself. Let's just say that I am not a fan of driving in Boston. Fortunately, I know the area around Mass General Hospital pretty well, so it didn't take me long to find the parking lot.

I remember walking into Mass Eye and Ear, and it being very strict. They made sure we were masked, our hands were sanitized, and there were only six people per elevator ride. Luckily for me, it was not busy the day I went in, and the waiting rooms were practically empty. Normally, it was the other way around.

When the surgery was done, I could hear out of both my ears. I was so proud. I could *actually* hear and understand what people were saying. It was a 40th birthday dream come true.

My theory on my hearing loss is that, for some reason, my ears never finished developing like they were supposed to while I was in my mother's womb. I was tested for hearing multiple times in school, but I was a smart girl, and they would miss my sneakiness. I knew which buttons they were touching. I was deaf throughout my life, and I had no idea until I was almost 40 years old. Can you believe that? I still can't to this day.

On March 27, 2020, I turned 40. My family was planning a surprise party for me. Due to COVID, the restaurant they had reserved had to cancel. This was the first time it hit me that the world was shutting down. I believe I was in denial the whole time before my birthday party was cancelled.

Who wants to cancel their 40th birthday party? I didn't. When I was a kid, something bad would always happen on my birthday, and 98% of the time, I would get sick, and no one would be able to come over. I only had one major birthday party when I was eleven or twelve, one that included both family and friends, and it was a lot of fun. Now, because of COVID, I had to cancel a major milestone.

I knew the world was on pause, but I had no idea how fast I would lose clients. I transitioned from a thriving pet-sitting business to one that was barely running. 90% of my clients didn't need me anymore, mainly because they were all working from home. I was down to 1-2 clients. I took some time off to ensure I didn't contract COVID. I didn't want to pass it on to my clients in any way. No one knew if they had it or not. Things seemed very vague at this time. It seemed that if you walked outside your house, you would catch it, regardless of whether you came into contact with other people or not.

Due to COVID, I had to put my business completely on hold. By June, I had given up and started walking for one client. I hadn't been out of the house in over three months, and I felt so tired of staying in my bedroom doing nothing. This walk reminded me that, even though it felt like the world was on pause, I was still here. Tired, bored, but still moving.

CHAPTER 10

Born to Flourish

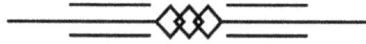

———=◆◇◆=———

In June of 2020, I decided to take a course to become a pet first-aid instructor. It was a wonderful addition to my business. It gave me something new to work on, and I was happy to take on the challenge.

A pet first-aid instructor was exactly what it sounded like. I would be able to teach anyone interested in pet safety, and I could teach them from anywhere. Pet first-aid is a must for professionals who work in the pet industry, like me. I loved the idea of it, and I was so excited about my new adventure.

I took a 3-day course to learn the skills I needed. After graduating, we received all the necessary information to teach the course. The name of my little company was Paws Fur Safety, and I couldn't wait to get started.

As soon as July came around, my clients were ready to go on vacation, and I was eager to have them back. Before anyone went on vacation, they had to test negative for COVID-19. I would be working for at least 1-2 clients around the 4th of July week, and it made me happy to get in the swing of things. I still only had one daily client, which was sad, but it was great to get out of the house and do what I loved.

Towards the end of summer, my mom and I talked about adopting a cat. I needed a best friend whom I could love daily. I initially wanted a kitten, but I was having the worst time finding one. I reached out to a Facebook friend who I knew worked at a rescue in New Hampshire, and she showed me a picture of a cat named Minnie. I fell in love with her before I met her.

When I finally saw her in person, she was the sweetest cat, sitting on my lap within minutes of meeting me. I believe I cried that day, and I told my friend I was going to take her home.

Minnie was 2 years old when I adopted her. She was an indoor/outdoor cat that, within two years before she was surrendered, had two successful litters of kittens. Her third litter didn't make it. She had fallen out of a second-story window and broken her left back leg. When this happened, the owner tried to put her down because they couldn't afford the surgery and didn't want a wobbling cat that couldn't walk for 6 to 8 weeks. From my understanding of her paperwork, Minnie was surrendered when she got pregnant the third time.

After having this cat for almost 5 years, I can confidently say she is the most amazing and sweetest cat you would ever meet. She greets anyone who walks in the door without judgment. She loves attention and being under the covers - that's where she is right now as I'm writing this chapter. It's her favorite place to be.

I believe that Minnie gave me the ability to love and care for something other than myself. I was missing something in my life, and in all reality, that was her. I love animals; it's who I am, and I would do anything for them, but Minnie is my child in cat form. I love her more than any animal I have ever met, and even more than any animal my parents have owned. She can be a pain in the neck at 5:30 a.m., but I don't mind - I'll always get up to take care of her. People may call her spoiled, but she's simply loved to the moon and back.

Now, let's get to the good part: the day I met the one guy who changed my life for the better.

I dated over the years, but honestly, no one ever quite piqued my interest. I didn't have anyone that I wanted to spend every day with. It was "Okay, I like you," and then I'd lose interest and move on.

Until I met him.

We met on eHarmony, a platform that differs slightly from other dating apps. They give you a test to make sure that you're a fit for the platform and its members. When I was a member, it worked in a way that you wanted a high match, around 90% or above. Ryan and I were 116%.

We started talking on eHarmony, and we clicked instantly. Our first phone call lasted almost an hour. He asked me out that night, with the date scheduled for two days later.

I remember our first date as if it were yesterday. It was six days before Christmas on December 19, 2020. We went to a restaurant that was about ten minutes away from my house. He was tall and handsome - two things that were checked off on my list. I asked if I could hug him, and he said yes. It was butterflies the moment we hugged. I was nervous, but I was comfortable. I felt like I met my best friend and we'd known each other for years.

We talked more than we ate, and then we went back to his place to watch TV because we didn't want the date to end. He was very respectable and wanted to take things slowly. I was more than okay with slow. We sat next to each other, and I remember struggling, trying not to touch his hand.

By the end of the first date, I went in for a kiss while he went in for a hug. It was awkward, but it was okay because it was a successful first date, and he asked to see me again.

Within a month, I saw him seventeen times and spent many nights at his place. We saw each other every couple of days just to make sure we weren't jumping in too fast. A little more than a month after we met, we became official and even announced our status on Facebook.

As the months went on, he met my mom, Andy, and Grace and her family. My mom knew he loved me from the moment she met him. We hadn't even said "I love you" until almost two months later. They adored him, and he became not only my significant other but a part of my family.

During this time, on Memorial Day weekend of 2021, I had my third surgery and ended up getting an Osia 2 for my right ear. It was great that I was able to connect both of my hearing aids together. The fun thing about hearing aids is that they work using Bluetooth, and I can listen to just about anything at any time. The tricky thing about having two different manufacturers of hearing aids was that they wouldn't sync together, which meant I couldn't listen to podcasts and audiobooks in the same ear. It got frustrating. Ryan didn't see me right after surgery, mostly because I was so tired, and I spent a lot of it sleeping when I wasn't with my family. I was overall exhausted and was barely even able to take a shower.

By June 2021, Minnie was a traveling cat. Ryan always wanted me to stay at his place longer, so I started bringing Minnie with me. This way, I was able to stay for the whole weekend and not go back and forth between his place and mine because I was constantly worrying about her. Let's say that Minnie was not made to travel; to this day, she hates being confined in a cat carrier.

The more Minnie was at Ryan's, the better and more comfortable she became. When it was time to leave, she would start hiding, so I would just go to work and leave her at his house. She loved having the space and enjoyed being with him.

By September, Minnie had her essentials moved in before I did. Ryan loved Minnie, and she trusted him. Not many people can pick up my cat and make her stay still for over a minute. Ryan could hold her forever. She cuddles, but she will not sit on someone's lap. I am Minnie's person, but it's obvious she loves Ryan just as much as I do.

On December 1st, 2021, I met with a psychiatrist to get tested for ADHD. I always suspected I had it because my mind was constantly going from one thing to the next, and I could never stop moving my hands. I could never sit still, jumping from one activity to another. I can't, even now. The best way to describe ADHD, as I've seen it described on TikTok, is that you have ten songs playing in your head at once, and you just can't stop. Medication helps the noise go away.

On December 20, 2021, I was diagnosed with combined ADHD. Combined ADHD means that I'm inattentive, hyperactive, and impulsive. If you know me, you may not think I'm hyperactive, but I am. Hyperactivity isn't always on the outside; it can be on the inside, too. I can get excited about a new project and work on it for hours, and then lose interest the next minute.

It took me almost two years to get on medication. The short-term medication made me angry. I had to take it twice a day, and I didn't like it. The other medication didn't make me feel like myself. I was having a hard time even writing this book. Did it help? Yes, but it was as if I lost a part of myself. It may have helped me be a little more focused and calm my brain down, but I didn't love myself as a person.

One thing I never thought would happen was that I would have to close my pet-sitting business. 80% of my clients were working from home. I didn't have many clients anymore, and I had two choices: either get a job or start my business over.

I was still living with my mom and stepdad at this point - it wasn't until January 2022 that I would move in with Ryan, so I couldn't afford to start over when my business was barely running. I applied for a few jobs and even tried working at a daycare with children. I stayed there for 2 days. It wasn't the kids who were the problem; it was that there was no training. I may be a self-starter who managed to complete all the courses, but I knew nothing about actually teaching kids.

Within a couple of days, I started my search again. I found a job at a cell phone store, and I applied right away. I loved technology and I still do. Apple products were my favorite. I would watch every WWDC (Apple's Worldwide Developer Conference) every year. My interview with the store owner lasted about two hours, mostly because we got along well and shared a decent amount in common. I was hired within a day or two and started work that next week, part-time, until I could give my pet-sitting clients notice that my last day would be January 28, 2022.

The first week of my job at the cell phone store, I found out that we lost my Nana. She was having surgery on her hip, and she didn't make it. It was recommended that she not have surgery because of her heart. She was 98 years old. She always told me that she would go in her sleep, and I believed her, so losing my nana while she was in surgery was not what I was expecting. My Nana was someone who loved to be in the spotlight. Not that she caused drama, she was just happiest when she was noticed and given attention.

My nana, Patricia Nolan Lebeaux, was a psych nurse, director of nursing, and teacher, who retired as a nursing home inspector. She lived in Sandwich, MA, for thirty years, then moved closer to us in her mid-eighties and decided to relocate to the south, closer to my Aunt and Uncle, in 2015. She passed away in Savannah, Georgia, in 2022.

I talked to Nana the day before, and she was in good spirits and ready for her hip surgery. I admired her a lot for that. My mom spent plenty of time with my grandfather, but my Nana became a single mom, raising five kids starting in 1961. Most of the parenting fell on my Nana's shoulders. She was the strongest woman I knew, besides my mom.

I made it through work that day and went home, where I cried. Ryan was on a well-deserved cruise with his brother, and he was due back in a couple of days. It was so hard to be alone during that time. Even though I had family nearby, I just wanted my Ryan to be home. He was just as heartbroken as I was. It was decided that our family would host a catholic memorial, and then we would bury her ashes up north in the summer.

She picked her burial plot a long time ago. She had always wanted her ashes to be buried in Massachusetts. We buried Nana on August 17, 2022. It was a sad day, but we did our best to make the most of it as a family. We loved her so much, and she's still missed very much to this day.

A day or two after we buried Nana's ashes, I wasn't feeling too well, but I went to work anyway. As the day went on, I started to feel worse and worse and asked to go home. I was feeling very hot. My co-workers thought that I had COVID, but no one wanted to jump to conclusions.

I went home, and I was in bed for so long. My COVID-19 test came back positive, and I had no idea what was happening. I took a stress dose of my prednisone and hoped I would be okay. Then came the vomiting. I am not someone who can easily make it to the toilet - it was either get sick or sleep, so I slept a lot. Ryan went to work, but he quickly realized he also wasn't feeling well, so he took a COVID-19 test at work. When it came back positive, he decided to head home to check on me and rest. At that point, I had been sleeping for close to 14 hours. He tried to get me to eat or drink something, but if I did, I immediately got sick. It was the worst I felt in a long time.

By Saturday, Ryan was starting to get worried about me. He drove me to urgent care for a hydration drip, but we had to go to a second location because our local urgent care didn't have the capability for IV. He had to drive me another 15 minutes, then he had to wait outside, while he himself was sick with COVID. He was patient throughout the entire process, waiting for me to recover. I was given Zofran for vomiting, and I started to feel much better. I was able to go back to work a few days later, still wearing a mask. It probably took me a week or longer to get better.

I met some of the best coworkers working at my job at the cell phone store. I made some great friends and I was happy there. I learned everything there was to know about cell phones. Learning technology is such a hard job. Not only did you need to understand it, but you also had to be able to solve problems quickly. I felt like we were constantly learning about new cell phones, tablets, and watch promotions. There were so many different devices on the market that I could tell you about each and every one of them and the deals that went with them. You had to stay focused and remember many different things. I tell you, working at a cell phone store is more challenging than you think. Yes, I got to play with new electronics all the time, but there was a lot of training and many different things we had to do.

I would say it was the job that was the most challenging, one that kept me on my toes even more than dog walking, but I loved it more than I could say. I stayed for a little under two years. I don't know why, but I seem to struggle with staying with a company for more than two years. My performance was great, but I was missing something.

I felt like I had a huge gaping hole in my gut, and working at a cell phone store just wasn't enough for me. I missed my time with my cat and my boyfriend. I missed working with animals more than anyone knew. Yes, I saw my cat, who's the best in the world, daily, but it just wasn't enough. I truly missed waking up at 6 a.m. to go feed a dog, feeling fulfilled by the end of the day. While there were great customers, they weren't always the best customers, and I didn't feel fulfilled when my shift was done.

I gave my two-week notice after going from full-time to part-time over the summer. I was only working Thursday through Sunday, reducing my hours from 40 to 29 a week. I began promoting my name in the pet-care industry and started freelancing for a friend in the same field. I was building my website and my business while working part-time. In late August, I gave my notice. My last day was to be September 16, 2023.

On September 2, 2023, I got a phone call I wasn't expecting. I was at work alone until the end of the day, and my sister called when I was with a customer. She asked if I could call back because it was an emergency. Andy had a stroke. He was at the hospital, but he was okay so far. My mom acted fast. He was standing, and all of a sudden, he wasn't. My mom got him up and called the ambulance, got him to a hospital in the next town over, and got him medication needed to stop the stroke right away.

I called my boss and told him that I had to go. I was having a hard time being there, and I just wanted to leave. He told me to wait for the other employee, and then a few minutes later, he called and told me I could lock up and head home.

I got home, and Ryan and I went to the hospital to see him. Andy came out with flying colors. He could talk and didn't lose much of his muscle mass. Because of my mom's quick thinking, he was completely fine. He didn't need surgery. Andy could go home in a few days.

We were all relieved that he was okay. Life moved on once he was good. He still goes to doctors' appointments, but he's in good shape now and has had no issues since his stroke.

Before I knew it, I was done at the cell phone store. I was sad to leave. I'm pretty sure I cried when I left, but at least I got to work with my favorite coworker on my last day. I was so happy that it was just the two of us that day.

Life moved on, and soon enough, I started helping my pet-sitter friend out pretty much full-time while building my clientele. It was great because I was working and feeling fulfilled every day. I even got home in time to make dinner and do housework.

Then, one day in late October 2023, I saw something on Facebook that changed my life. A publisher was looking for authors, and if you were accepted, you could become a published author. I was accepted, and even though this book is being published almost a year after the first publication date, I am beyond proud that I chose to stay with it.

I've been writing this book since November 2023. It's been a whirlwind of emotions and writer's block to get where I am today. The title Born to Flourish came to me when I was on a dog walk in 2018. At first, I thought it would be a blog title about Panhypopituitarism, but when this project came around, I knew it was the perfect title for my book.

This was the right project for me. I've always loved writing, and being a published author was just the icing on the cake.

To update all my readers, I have been with Ryan for almost four and a half years, and Minnie is still a solo cat. Ryan did promise me that if I sold at least 100 books, I could get Minnie a friend.

I am running Nancy's Cat Care full time. I changed to cats because I'm more of a cat person than a dog person. I still have more dog clients than cat clients, but I decided to focus on cats due to the anxiety I experience from walking reactive dogs. Not all dogs are bad, but I have been in enough scary situations, and I just don't want to be the person who fears walking dogs. I walk a few that I trust, but walking a dog that I haven't built a relationship with is hard for me.

All this to say, life is good and I'm beyond happy where I am today and what I have built over the last 45 years. It may not be perfect, but I'm proud of the person I have become.

Who knows what I'll be up to a year from now? Maybe I'll write more books, or maybe I won't. If you want to find out what I'm currently up to go to my website msnancyhill.com.

As I end this book, I'm reminded of how far I've come - I've not only defied my teacher's expectations and graduated high school, but I've also become a published author. Life is surprising and full of twists and turns. I used to think having panhypopituitarism was an inescapable prison, but now I see that you can still have a great life despite it.

I don't know what the future holds, but I'm sure of one thing: I was born to flourish.

Acknowledgements

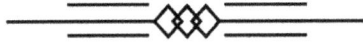

Thank you to the love of my life, Scott Bauman, for supporting me throughout this journey and being the best partner anyone could ask for. Your encouragement has kept me going throughout this process. I love you.

To Minnie: You may just be a cat, but at seven years old, you are the reason I wake up every morning. I have to wake up because if I don't, you will find a way to annoy me. Your presence brings joy and love into our lives. We love you.

To my mom, Rosemary Southwick: Thank you for always fighting for me. I wouldn't have made it without your perseverance and the belief that I was normal; I just had to find my way. Again, if you want to read about the first year of my life, buy her book, *If They'd Only Listen*.

To Randy: Thank you for always pushing me to do my best. Your belief in me, encouragement, and steady support have meant more than I can ever express.

To Jamie, Steve, Von, and Veanna: Thank you for always believing in me and cheering me on throughout this process. I couldn't have written this book without your love and support.

To the rest of my family and friends who knew I was going through this process: Your collective belief in me and unwavering support were the fuel that kept me going. This book is as much yours as it is mine. Thank you for being there every step of the way.

To my nana, who is no longer with us: You were on my mind while I wrote this book. I know you would be beyond proud of me. I know you'll be shouting from the rooftops in heaven. I love you.

To my Facebook group, Congenital Panhypopituitarism: Over the last ten years, we have built an unbelievable family of over 716 members and growing. Your support and shared experiences have been invaluable to me. I couldn't have done this without every one of you.

To the **She Rises Studios family**: This book wouldn't have happened without every single one of you. You helped me realize my dreams and pushed me to write it. Born to Flourish would've been in my mind for another ten years if it weren't for your team.

To everyone mentioned here, and those whose impact is felt even if not named, thank you for shaping the person I am and for being part of this journey. This book is as much yours as it is mine.

About the Author

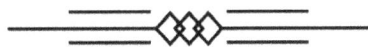

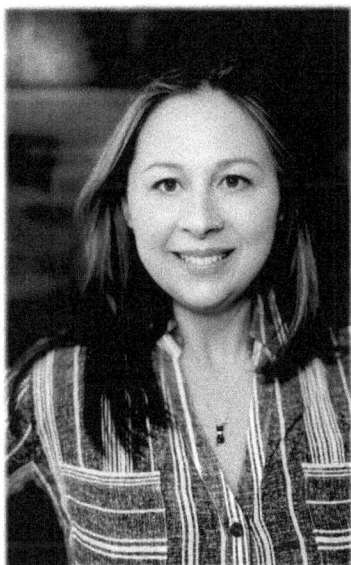

Nancy Hill is a 45-year-old female who was diagnosed with a rare disease called Panhypopituitarism when she was ten days old in 1980. She is the author of Born to Flourish: My Journey to Becoming Panhypopituitarism Strong.

Nancy has a Facebook group of over 700 members called Congenital Panhypopituitarism. She is launching her first podcast, Empowered by Rare, which features stories of patients with rare diseases. To learn more about Nancy's upcoming projects, please visit her website, msnancyhill.com.

LinkedIn: https://www.linkedin.com/in/nancy-hill/
Facebook: https://facebook.com/msnancyhill
Instagram: http://instagram.com/msnancyhill
Websites: http://msnancyhill.com

www.ingramcontent.com/pod-product-compliance
Lightning Source LLC
Chambersburg PA
CBHW060237030426
42335CB00014B/1504